To Jan Nov 11,

Best wishes

Cellular and Humoral Immunotherapy and Apheresis

Cellular and Humoral Immunotherapy and Apheresis

Editors

Ronald A. Sacher, MD, FRCP(C)
Professor of Medicine and Pathology
Director of Transfusion Medicine
Georgetown University Medical Center
Washington, District of Columbia

Daniel B. Brubaker, DO
Chief Executive Officer
Scientific Director
Spokane and Inland Empire Blood Bank
Spokane, Washington

Duke O. Kasprisin, MD
Chief Medical Officer
American Red Cross Blood Services
Oklahoma Region
Tulsa, Oklahoma

Leo J. McCarthy, MD
Professor of Pathology and Medicine
Director of Transfusion Medicine
Indiana University Medical Center
Indianapolis, Indiana

Special thanks are extended to Fenwal Division—Baxter Healthcare Corporation for their generous support of the AABB's workshop, "Cellular and Humoral Immunotherapy and Apheresis." We are grateful for their contribution to the success of this educational activity.

American Association of Blood Banks
Arlington, Virginia
1991

American Association of Blood Banks   ISBN NO. 1-56395-001-4
1117 North 19th Street, Suite 600   Printed in the United States
Arlington, Virginia 22209

Library of Congress Cataloging-in-Publication Data

Cellular and humoral immunotherapy and apheresis/
editors, Ronald A. Sacher ... [et al.].
p. cm.
Prepared for use at an American Association of Blood Banks workshop.
Includes bibliographical references and index.
ISBN 1-56395-001-4
1. Immunotherapy. 2. Hemapheresis. 3. Cancer—Immunotherapy.
4. Bone marrow—Transplantation. I. Sacher, Ronald R.
II. American Association of Blood Banks.
[DNLM: 1. Blood Component Removal—methods. 2. Immunity, Cellular.
3. Immunotherapy, Adoptive—methods. 4. Neoplasms—therapy. QW 940 C393]
RM275.C45 1991
615'.39—dc20
DNLM/DLC
for Library of Congress
91-32912
CIP

Technical/Scientific Workshops Committee

Dennis M. Smith, Jr., MD, Chairman

Michael L. Baldwin, MBA, MT(ASCP)SBB
Alice Reynolds Barr, SBB(ASCP)
Daniel B. Brubaker, DO
Katherine B. Carlson, MT(ASCP)SBB
Morris R. Dixon, MS, MT(ASCP)SBB
Frances L. Gibbs, MS, MT(ASCP)SBB
Christina A. Kasprisin, MS, RN
Sanford R. Kurtz, MD
Barbara Laird-Fryer, MT(ASCP)SBB
Judith S. Levitt, MT(ASCP)SBB
Leo J. McCarthy, MD
JoAnn M. Moulds, PhD
Ronald A. Sacher, MD
Phyllis Unger, MT(ASCP)SBB
Robert G. Westphal, MD
Susan M. Wilson, MT(ASCP)SBB
Laura Lee Woods, MS, MT(ASCP)SBB

Contents

Foreword

Apheresis continues its increasingly important role in modern transfusion medicine, not only for platelet collection and therapeutic procedures, but also for the collection of bone marrow stem cells for transplantation and immune cells for modulation. New and expanding immunologic concepts require a basic understanding of the immune regulatory mechanisms for all those applying apheresis to donors and especially patients. Major developments in the immune regulating network are summarized as are the current indications for apheresis. The cellular aspects of molecular recognition and immunoregulation are thoroughly discussed and provide invaluable information.

Peripheral stem cell collection has benefitted autologous bone marrow transplant patients by providing sufficient numbers of stem cells for engraftment. It is now used for many patients whose marrows are involved with neoplasms or are otherwise unacceptable for aspiration. The indications and techniques for collecting peripheral blood stem cells are discussed. Circulating immune cells can also be collected and then treated with lymphokines, which activate their ability to kill tumor cells. Extracorporeal photopheresis, licensed for treating cutaneous T-cell lymphomas, is being evaluated in the treatment of various immune diseases and transplantation since it modulates the immune system.

This entire field is expanding very rapidly and this book provides an excellent and concise up-to-date review of the current "state of the art" and concludes with the exciting future of cellular immunotherapy as it applies to bone marrow transplantation and cancer.

Daniel B. Brubaker, DO
Duke O. Kasprisin, MD
Leo J. McCarthy, MD
Ronald A. Sacher, MD, FRCP(C)
Editors

In: Sacher RA, Brubaker DB, Kasprisin DO and McCarthy LJ, eds.
Cellular and Humoral Immunotherapy and Apheresis
Arlington, VA: American Association of Blood Banks, 1991

1

Immunoglobulin Biology and Therapeutic Mechanisms Involved in Immunoglobulin Therapy

Alan D. Schreiber, MD; Milton D. Rossman, MD;
and Arnold I. Levinson, MD

FOR MANY YEARS IMMUNE serum globulin has been used as replacement therapy in patients with immunoglobulin deficiency. The product was obtained by fractionation of pooled human plasma and was administered by intramuscular injection. The intravenous use of intramuscular immunoglobulin was limited by side effects that included chills, fever and hypotension. In the 1970's investigators developed intravenous immunoglobulin (IVIG) preparations with the intent to improve immunoglobulin replacement therapy in patients with immunodeficiency.

Mechanisms of Action of Immunoglobulin Therapy

The use of IVIG in immune thrombocytopenic purpura (ITP) and other noninfectious diseases, such as immunohematologic disorders, was first noted in the 1980's.[1] Under these circumstances, IVIG was given in considerably higher doses than those required for the prophylaxis of infection. Intravenous immunoglobulin therapy was shown to be effective in the treatment of both adults and children with ITP; on occasion, its effect was observed to be sustained.[2] The success of IVIG in the treatment of ITP led

Alan D. Schreiber, MD, Professor of Medicine, Chairman of the Graduate Group in Immunology and Assistant Dean for Research, School of Medicine, University of Pennsylvania, Milton D. Rossman, MD, Associate Professor of Medicine, School of Medicine, University of Pennsylvania; and Arnold I. Levinson, MD, Associate Professor of Medicine, Department of Medicine, School of Medicine, University of Pennsylvania, Philadelphia, Pennsylvania to its use in other potentially immune disorders. These disorders included those involving acquired inhibitors of coagulation factors, neonatal alloimmune thrombocytopenic purpura, posttransfusion purpura, autoimmune hemolytic anemia, autoimmune pancytopenia, thrombotic thrombocytopenic purpura and refractoriness to platelet transfusions due to alloantibodies.[3]

Effects on Immune Clearance

Intravenous immunoglobulin therapy is effective in a large number of patients with ITP and this treatment is indicated when thrombocytopenia is severe and life-threatening, particularly in the setting of unresponsiveness to glucocorticoid therapy.[4-7,9] Therapy is most effective in ITP and other conditions that involve the autoantibody-induced destruction of blood cells when compared to other disorders such as therapy for acquired inhibitors of Factor VIII and Factor IX.

Although there have been good studies to define the mechanism of the early effect of IVIG in ITP, there has been considerably less work in understanding the long-term response to this therapy. The major mechanisms by which IVIG therapy has been shown to be effective include the following:

1. The clearance of antibody-coated cells from the circulation is inhibited.[4]
2. The deposition on the cell surface of biologically active fragments of complement is inhibited.[7]
3. Anti-idiotypic antibodies present in IVIG preparations may react with and interfere with the function of autoantibodies responsible for the immune clearance or immune damage. Anti-idiotypic antibodies in IVIG preparations may also react with idiotypes on B lymphocytes or T lymphocytes and in that manner interfere with the autoimmune response.[8]
4. Antibodies reactive with red blood cell antigens, such as ABO or Rh antigens, present in IVIG preparations may enhance the clearance of autologous red cells and in that manner inhibit macrophage-mediated clearance of autoantibody opsonized cells.[6]

The Role of Macrophages

The most compelling studies are those indicating that IVIG interferes with the clearance of antibody-coated cells. It has been suggested that small quantities of IgG aggregates found in IVIG preparations or even monomeric IgG may be responsible for this effect. Macrophages express a wide range of Fcγ receptors, which are encoded by seven different genes, thus far described. These genes encode for Fcγ receptor proteins on the cell surface.

The Human Fcγ Receptors

At least three biochemically distinct Fcγ receptors have been described on human cells, and each appears to be present on the surface of human macrophages. These receptors have been designated FcγRI (CD 64), FcγRII (CD 32) and FcγRIII (CD 16). They are membrane glycoproteins with extracellular domains that contain immunoglobulin-like regions. Therefore, they are members of the immunoglobulin gene superfamily. They appear to be located on human chromosome 1 and may have arisen from gene duplication.

Fcγ Receptor FcγRI

FcγRI (CD 64) was first isolated from the U-937 human monocyte/macrophage cell line by Anderson using IgG-Sepharose affinity chromatography. These studies led to the identification of FcγRI as a 72,000-kDa glycoprotein that has a 40,000 molecular weight protein core following digestion with glycosidase.[10] Equilibrium binding studies with monomeric IgG indicated that human FcγRI is capable of binding monomeric IgG with high affinity, association constant equal to $1 \times 10^8 M^{-1}$ [11-17] and that FcγRI binds the human IgG subclasses IgG1 and IgG3 with higher affinity than subclasses IgG2 and IgG4.[18-22] Similar FcγRI subclass specificity appears to be present on inflammatory peritoneal macrophages[21] and the monocyte cell line U-937.[15]

The Fc domain that is recognized by FcγRI has now been defined and has been localized to the IgG CH2 domain. One additional means to identify FcγRI has been to utilize the specificity expressed for mouse immunoglobulin of a specific subclass, a characteristic of the human Fcγ receptors. FcγRI binds relatively specifically to monomeric mouse IgG of the subclass IgG2a. Furthermore, several monoclonal antibodies have thus far been isolated that recognize epitopes on FcγRI.[23-25] The gene for human FcγRI has recently been cloned.[20] The extracellular region of FcγRI consists of three immunoglobulin-like domains, two of which share homology with the other Fcγ receptors. This unique third domain may be responsible for the ability of FcγRI to bind monomeric IgG and to exhibit high affinity. Transfection studies in COS cells reveals a single species of approximately 70 kDa. Northern blot analysis with an FcγRI DNA probe demonstrates a single 1.7 kb RNA transcript in monocytes and placental macrophages, although this is not a consistent finding in all fresh monocytes. In U-937 cells, both a 1.7 kb and 1.6 kb transcript has been noted, each of which increased following incubation of U-937 cells with γ-interferon. Three polymorphisms have been observed among FcγRI cDNAs obtained from a single patient, which has led to the suggestion that there may be more than one gene encoding FcγRI. The predicted polypeptide sequence shows a hydrophobic signal sequence, a 21-residue hydrophobic transmembrane region and a charged cytoplasmic domain.

Our data indicate that both γ-interferon and glucocorticoids can modulate the expression of FcγRI on U-937 cells.[12,26-29] In addition, Northern blot analysis reveals that the steady state levels of mRNA are influenced by these two mediators.[28-30] Our hypothesis is that the interaction of glucocorticoid hormone with its receptor (a DNA binding protein) may decrease FcγRI mRNA levels by inducing a gene regulatory protein that differentially affects the transcription of FcγRI. Alternatively, glucocorticoid hormone interaction with its DNA binding protein receptor may lead to an association with FcγRI DNA. This, in turn, could regulate the binding and/or activation of FcγRI RNA polymerase. In the case of glucocorticoids one possibility is that binding or activation of RNA polymerase to FcγRI DNA is inhibited. With γ-interferon, the effect of RNA polymerase on FcγRI transcription may be enhanced.

As noted, FcγRI has a relatively high affinity for monomeric IgG. Since monocytes and macrophages are exposed to high concentrations (5-10 mg/mL) of circulating IgG, under most circumstances FcγRI is likely saturated with IgG monomer. Thus, the raison d'etre for FcγRI is at present uncertain. However, a compelling argument for the importance of FcγRI can be made by the ease with which the number and the density of these surface receptors can be modulated. γ-interferon will increase both the number and the surface density of FcγRI on monocytes.[26,30-31] An increased number of FcγRI appears within 8-12 hours and persists for at least 7 days. The increase in FcγRI due to γ-interferon has been demonstrated both by immunofluorescent and monomeric IgG binding studies. α-interferon and β-interferon appear to have little or no effect on macrophage FcγRI.[32] In contrast, glucocorticoid hormones substantially inhibit the expression of FcγRI on U-937 cells; however, glucocorticoids are less effective in inhibiting FcγRI on monocytes.[26,33] Paradoxically, glucocorticoids and γ-interferon appear to have a synergistic effect in increasing FcγRI on human monocytes, but have opposite effects on the expression and ligand binding capacity of FcγRI on the monocyte cell line U-937.[26,29,33]

Fcγ Receptor FcγRII

FcγRII (CD32) was initially isolated from the U-937 cell line using affinity chromatography. As with FcγRI, FcγRII was immunoprecipitated with an anti-Fcγ receptor antibody raised in rabbits by immunization with affinity-purified Fcγ binding protein. A monoclonal antibody was subsequently observed to bind to an epitope associated with the FcγRII ligand binding site.[34] This antibody immunoprecipitated a 40,000-kDa protein present on monocytes, neutrophils, platelets, B cells and the K562 cell line.[34] FcγRII does not bind monomeric IgG and binds oligomeric IgG with low affinity. The association constant of FcγRII for trimeric IgG is ~ $1 \times 10^7 M^{-1}$.[33-37] Characterization of FcγRII on human macrophages with murine immunoglobulin isotypes revealed that subclasses IgG1 and IgG2b bind to FcγRII with relative specificity.[36] On U-937 cells, aggregates of mouse IgG2b demonstrated enhanced binding to FcγRII under conditions of low ionic strength and low temperature. We have observed that similar conditions facilitate human oligomeric IgG binding to platelets and HEL cells, which express FcγRII as their only Fcγ receptor.[37]

We have observed that at normal ionic strength and at 37 C a low affinity receptor for trimeric IgG can be detected on in vitro cultured monocytes and freshly isolated alveolar macrophages.[38] We have demonstrated that this low affinity binding site for trimeric IgG on macrophages appears to represent FcγRII, since it is specifically inhibited by anti-FcγRII. A similar low affinity binding site for dimeric IgG, perhaps due to FcγRII, had been observed on inflammatory peritoneal macrophages[21] and monocytes cultured in vitro for 7 days.[39] In contrast, freshly isolated blood monocytes and U-937 cells, despite expressing abundant FcγRII protein, do not express a low affinity dimeric or trimeric IgG binding site.[40] This suggests that posttranslational modifications are involved in the functional expression of FcγRII. We have noted that exposure of monocytes to cold temperatures (4 C) further increases the expression of monocyte FcγRII.[40]

Despite the relative inability of FcγRII on monocytes to bind oligomers of human IgG under physiologic conditions, FcγRII has an important role in the human T-cell proliferative response to mouse IgG1 anti-T cell antibodies.[41] Monocytes from approximately 30% of normal individuals fail to stimulate T-cell proliferation (nonresponders) in the presence of IgG1 anti-T cell antibody.[42] When samples of purified monocyte FcγRII from responder and nonresponder individuals were compared, no difference in electrophoretic mobility on sodium dodecylsulphate-polyacrylamide gel electropheresis (SDS-PAGE) was observed.[41] However, different patterns were observed after isoelectric focusing. FcγRII from nonresponder individuals had multiple regularly spaced bands, while FcγRII from responders revealed either multiple regularly spaced bands asynchronous from those of nonresponders or multiple bands that were a combination of each pattern. The data suggest that FcγRII is encoded by a single gene with two alleles that differ in their interaction with IgG1.

FcγRII was the first human Fcγ receptor gene cloned.[43-45] Subsequent to the original publications, FcγRII clones have been reported by other laboratories including our own.[46] It appears that FcγRII is encoded by at least three genes (FcγRIIA, FcγRIIB and FcγRIIC). The extracellular domains encoded by the isolated clones are closely related to the extracellular domains of FcγRI and FcγRIII and to the extracellular domains of the analogous murine 2b/1β Fcγ receptor. Similarly, the transmembrane domain of FcγRII is homologous to that of murine FcγRIIβ. Differences exist in the transmembrane region and considerable differences exist in the intracellular domain of the FcγRII cDNAs when compared to those of FcγRI and FcγRIII. The cytoplasmic domain contains both neutral and hydrophobic residues. The differences in the cytoplasmic domains suggest that intracellular signalling events may differ considerably among these three human Fcγ receptors. Northern blot analysis reveals two major transcripts of 2.4 and 1.6 kb in most of the cells thus far examined that express FcγRII. Work on the genomic structure of FcγRII has begun, but is not yet complete.

FcγRII is the only Fcγ receptor present on human platelets. We have cloned FcγRII from a cDNA library prepared from the megakaryocyte/platelet-like cell line HEL.[46] One of our FcγRII cDNA clones is of particular note. This clone, 2.1 kb in size, is identical to published sequences in the extracellular region, but has an important difference downstream. There is an in-frame deletion of 123 nucleotides, which eliminates the DNA for the entire transmembrane region, suggesting alternative splicing of the primary transcript that removes this specific sequence. The 2.1 kb clone does not share structural features with FcγRI or FcγRIII, based on nucleotide and amino acid sequence comparison. This clone may encode for a soluble form of FcγRII, and using the polymerase chain reaction we have noted that it is identified in platelet, monocyte, HEL cell and U-937 cell FcγRII mRNA.[46]

The precise function of FcγRII on monocytes and macrophages is uncertain. We have discussed the conditions involved in FcγRII-mediated IgG ligand binding above. Monocyte FcγRII can induce IgG antibody-induced cell-mediated cytotoxicity.[47] Furthermore, it appears that crosslinking of FcγRII is necessary for its activation. A rise in intracellular calcium can be induced in U-937 cells and monocytes by both intact IgG1 and anti-FcγRII.[48] This may require a tripartite crosslinking of Fc and $F(ab')_2$, since calcium mobilization does not occur with $F(ab')_2$ fragments in the absence of the Fc domain.[48] In addition, superoxide production after FcγRII crosslinking has been noted, but only after γ-interferon priming of U-937 cells or monocytes. This may reflect intracellular alterations directly due to γ-interferon, rather than a γ-interferon effect on FcγRII. The hierarchy of human IgG subclass binding to FcγRII appears to be IgG1 > IgG2 ≥ IgG4 ≥ IgG3. These data have been derived from radiolabeled IgG ligand binding studies with FcγRII transfected COS cells.[45]

FcγRII expression can be regulated by granulocyte-macrophage colony-stimulating factor (GM-CSF) on U-937 cells, an effect that requires protein synthesis.[35] We have observed a substantial stimulatory effect of GM-CSF on human monocyte FcγRII (Rossman MD et al, unpublished observations). GM-CSF and γ-interferon also have been noted to increase FcγRII protein expression on U-937 cells.[29,35] Northern blot analysis reveals that U-937 cells treated with interferon-γ exhibit a 2.5-fold increase in FcγRII mRNA levels that is maximal at 14 hours and declines to 1.4-fold over baseline by 48 hours of incubation.[29] Treatment with glucocorticoids (dexamethasone) induces a small, but significant, decrease in FcγRII protein; dexamethasone is also able to inhibit by 20-60% the induction of FcγRII by γ-interferon. Modulation by dexamethasone and γ-interferon of FcγRII protein expression on U-937 cells is markedly different from that of FcγRI in both magnitude and kinetics.[29] γ-interferon treatment increases FcγRII expression by 240% at 16 hours, and FcγRII remains elevated through 48 hours. In contrast, expression of FcγRII protein on U-937 cells is increased 56-72% after 16-24 hours of γ-interferon treatment and is minimal after 48 hours of incubation. Thus, the modulation of FcγRII on U-937 cells is at least in part due to changes in steady state levels of FcγRII mRNA. We have recently shown that this is due to an effect on FcγRII transcription (Comber PG et al, unpublished observations). Furthermore, the difference between the magnitude of the changes in FcγRII mRNA and protein suggests that some translational or posttranslational control is involved in regulating the expression of FcγRII. Since FcγRI and FcγRII bind related ligands, mediate similar functions and appear to have similar changes in mRNA levels following γ-interferon treatment, it is possible the transcription of both genes is coordinately regulated. Isolation of the genomic sequences for FcγRI and FcγRII and analysis of 5'- and 3'-flanking sequences are being pursued to identify any common potential regulatory sequences.

Fcγ Receptor FcγRIII

A third Fcγ receptor has been identified (FcγRIII or CD 16) that is present on tissue macrophages, neutrophils and natural killer (NK) cells. This receptor has a low affinity for IgG and binds human IgG1 and IgG3 more effectively than IgG2 and IgG4. When isolated by immunoprecipitation, FcγRIII has a broad electrophoretic mobility on SDS-PAGE (51,000-73,000 Mr). FcγRIII appears on monocytes after in vitro culture for 1-2 weeks and has been identified on freshly isolated peritoneal and alveolar macrophages.[49-51] FcγRIII is not detectable on U-937 cells or on uninduced HL-60 cells.

Several different monoclonal antibodies (3G8, 4F7, B73.1, Leu-11a,b and VEP-13) have been prepared that react with FcγRIII. The monoclonal antibodies against FcγRIII are directed toward different epitopes and vary in their capacity to inhibit IgG binding. On neutrophils, it has been shown that the blood group antigen NA1 and NA2 neutrophils represent alloantigens of FcγRIII.[52] Several different classes of anti-FcγRIII monoclonal antibodies have been identified based on their reactivity with NA1 and NA2 on neutrophils and NK cells.[53]

FcγRIII on neutrophils appears to be a phosphatidylinositol (PI)-anchored protein since the expression of FcγRIII is markedly diminished on neutrophils from patients with paroxysmal nocturnal hemoglobinuria (PNH), a disorder in which the expression of PI-anchored proteins is diminished (also see below).[54] In addition, treatment of normal neutrophils with glycosyl-PI-specific phospholipase C, an enzyme that disrupts PI linkages, reduces the expression of FcγRIII. Evidence that FcγRIII on neutrophils differs from FcγRIII on macrophages initially was derived from immunoprecipitation studies with the anti-FcγRIII monoclonal antibody 3G8.[49-50] Neutrophil immunoprecipitated FcγRIII has a broader electrophoretic mobility on SDS-PAGE than does FcγRIII isolated from *in vitro* cultured monocytes. In addition, after digestion with N-glycanase, neutrophil FcγRIII is cleaved to a 33,000 M_r protein core, while the in vitro cultured monocyte protein is not altered by N-glycanase and is a 55,000 Mr molecule.

FcγRIII has been cloned by Seed and co-workers, the same laboratory that cloned the genes for FcγRI and FcγRII.[55] These investigators employed a cDNA library from human placenta, presumably a source of monocytes and macrophages, and their transcripts. The data indicated that the extracellular domain of FcγRIII is closely homologous to that of FcγRI and FcγRII. However, in contrast to FcγRII, which bears greatest homology to the murine FcγRIIβ gene, FcγRIII is most homologous with the α form of the murine FcγRII gene. The extracellular domain of FcγRIII ends in a short 200 to 220-residue hydrophobic domain followed by four hydrophobic residues, of which one is charged. A similar structure and a similar hydrophobicity profile of the predicted amino acid sequence are characteristic of membrane proteins bearing a glycosyl-PI-phospholipid (P-I) linkage. This indicates that FcγRIII is a phospholipid anchored protein on at least some human cells in which it is expressed. In fact, it has been established that FcγRIII on human granulocytes and NK cells is at least in part P-I linked (see above). This distinguishes FcγRIII from FcγRI and FcγRII, which are not P-I linked.

It has been determined from our studies and those of others that FcγRIII on tissue macrophages is not a P-I linked molecule.[56] Patients with PNH have a deficiency in P-I linked proteins and their granulocytes are substantially deficient in FcγRIII. Nevertheless, it has been our experience and the experience of others that patients with PNH do not have a substantial increase in their incidence of infection. This may be due to active FcγRI and/or FcγRII function in host defense in these patients. Alternatively, FcγRIII may not be uniformly deficient in these patients and their macrophages, as opposed to their neutrophils, may express FcγRIII. The data indicate that FcγRIII is present on cells of the monocyte/macrophage binding in PNH, as well as normal individuals, as a conventional transmembrane non-P-I linked form of FcγRIII.[56]

Because FcγRIII is not abundant on freshly isolated monocytes, there have only been limited studies to define the function of FcγRIII on human macrophages. Clarkson et al employed the anti-FcγRIII monoclonal antibody 3G8 to inhibit the clearance of IgG-coated platelets in immune thrombocytopenic purpura.[57] Since the clearance of platelets in immune thrombocytopenia is mediated by splenic macrophage Fcγ receptors, the rise in platelet count after infusion of anti-FcγRIII is probably due to inhibition of immune clearance by these macrophage receptors. Thus, FcγRIII likely plays an important role in phagocytosis by tissue macrophages.

Monocytes and alveolar macrophages grown in the presence of fibroblast supernatant express increased levels of FcγRIII.[51] On the other hand, steroids and γ-interferon do not appear to alter the expression of FcγRIII in vitro.[33] We have observed that M-CSF and serum factors play a role in regulating the expression of FcγRIII on human monocytes/macrophages.

Summary

In summary, human macrophage Fcγ receptors are a heterogeneous group of glycoproteins, of which three distinct biochemical entities have been defined. With the cloning of the human Fcγ receptor genes and their biochemical characterization, emphasis will now focus on their likely diverse functions in host defense, immune complex recognition and intracellular signaling. In addition, the further characterization of soluble Fcγ receptors and their potential immunoregulatory significance will become an increasing area of focus and may illuminate the mechanism by which IVIG is effective.

However as was discussed above, it is now apparent that these Fcγ receptors do differ in their function. FcγRI, for example, is the only Fcγ receptor that binds monomeric IgG and it does so with high affinity. FcγRII and FcγRIII only recognize polyvalent IgG and, thus, only bind IgG aggregates or IgG-containing immune complexes. There are data that suggest that FcγRIII and FcγRII are the most important macrophage Fcγ receptors involved in the clearance of IgG-coated cells. However, to date it is still uncertain which Fcγ receptors are modulated by IVIG therapy in a manner that decreases the detection of IgG-coated cells, eg, IgG-sensitized platelets in ITP. It is of interest that this mechanism of action is one mechanism by which glucocorticoids exert their therapeutic efficacy in ITP. Glucocorticoids have been shown to interfere with macrophage Fcγ receptor function and expression in vivo. In fact, intravenous glucocorticoids have been shown to decrease the number of Fcγ receptors expressed on the cell surface and, therefore, to decrease the binding of IgG-coated cells to these receptors on the macrophage surface. This process occurs effectively with splenic macrophages. In ITP and IgG-induced immune hemolytic anemia, splenic macrophages play the major role in the clearance of IgG-sensitized cells.

Additional Immunomodulatory Properties of Immunoglobulin Therapy

The Effects of Complement-Dependent Immune Damage of Cells and Tissues

Another potential mechanism of action of IVIG that warrants some discussion is the interference of the deposition of biologically active fragments of complement onto the immune complex. This has been studied most effectively with red blood cells where IVIG has been shown to inhibit the deposition of C3b and C4b.[7,58]

Activation of complement often leads to the binding of complement components to individual immunoglobulin molecules. For example, C3 has been shown to bind to the Fc fragment of IgG in the form of a C3b-IgG complex. The C3b-IgG complex has new properties that differ from either IgG or C3b alone and the complex can then interact with two receptors on phagocytic cells, the complement receptor CR1, which binds C3b, and an Fcγ receptor. Particles opsonized with C3b-IgG interact with both receptors and are phagocytized rapidly. Bacteria coated with immunoglobulin and then incubated in serum have C3b deposited on their surface, which in many instances is bound to the IgG molecules. For example, 30% of the C3b deposited on antibody-coated pneumococci is bound not to the pneumococcal surface but to the coating immunoglobulin. It has been suggested that IVIG may act as a receptor for activated complement components, preventing their attachment to targets.

Experiments have been conducted to ascertain the site in the complement cascade at which IVIG acts to block complement action. As mentioned, C3b deposition on targets is inhibited by the presence of IVIG. C4 is a similar molecule with a similar thiolester structure and mechanism of action. C4b deposition on targets is inhibited by IVIG and the dose response curves of inhibition are superimposable for C3 and C4, suggesting that the mechanism of effect is similar. The latter studies have, thus far, been most effectively performed in animal models.

Modulation of Autoimmune Response Through the Interaction With Immune/Idiotype Networks

In acquired anti-Factor VIII disease, there are anti-idiotypic antibodies in IVIG that bind to idiotypes carried by pathogenic autoantibodies, thus neutralizing their effect. Sultan et al have[59] also demonstrated that IVIG preparations contain anti-idiotypic antibodies against the idiotypic determinants on a variety of other disease-associated autoantibodies, including anti-DNA, antithyroglobulin, anti-intrinsic factor and anti peripheral nerve autoantibodies. He further suggests that polyvalent passive IVIG may provide deficient regulatory idiotypic antibodies, implying that some of the therapeutic success with IVIG may be as a result of network regulation of immune responses. Thus, anti-idiotypic antibodies in IVIG preparation may also react with idiotypes on B lymphocytes or T lymphocytes, and in that manner interfere with the immune response.

Summary

In summary, there are several possible mechanisms involved in the response to immunoglobulin therapy. There is compelling evidence for an effect on macrophage Fcγ receptor expression. There is evidence for interference with C4b and C3b deposition on the immune complex. Finally, in some systems there is evidence for anti-idiotypic antibody interference with the production or action of the autoantibody.

Acknowledgment

The authors thank Ms. Ruth Rowan for her excellent assistance in preparing this manuscript for publication.

References

1. Imbach P, Barandun S, d'Apuzzo V, et al. High-dose intravenous gammaglobulin for idiopathic thrombocytopenic purpura in childhood. Lancet 1981;1:1228-31.
2. Bussel JB. The use of intravenous gamma globulin in idiopathic thrombocytopenic purpura (a review). Clin Imunol Immunopathol 1989;53:S147-55.
3. Berkman SA, Lee ML, Gale RP. Clinical uses of intravenous gamma globulin. Semin Hematol 1988;25:140-58.
4. Kurlander RJ, Ellison DM, Hall J. The blockade of Fc receptor-mediated clearance of immune complexes in vivo by monoclonal antibody (2.4G2) directed against Fc receptors on murine leukocytes. J Immunol 1984:133:855-62.
5. Fehr J, Hoffman V, Kappeler U. Transient reversal of thrombocytopenic purpura by high dose intravenous gamma globulin. N Engl Med 1982;306:1254-8.
6. Kimberly RP, Salmon JE, Bussel JB, et al. Modulation of mononuclear phagocyte function by intravenous gamma-globulin. J Immunol 1984;132:745-50.
7. Basta M, Langlois PF, Marques M, et al. High-dose intravenous immunoglobulin modifies complement-mediated in vivo clearance. Blood 1989;74:326-33.

8. Rossi F, Sultan Y, Kazatchkine MD. Spontaneous and therapeutic suppression of autoimmune response to factor VIII by anti-idiotypic antibodies. In: Morrell AA, Nydeger UE, eds. Clinical use of intravenous immunoglobulin. San Diego, CA: Academic, 1986:421.

9. Basta M, Kirshbom P, Frank MM, Fries LF. Mechanism of therapeutic effect of high-dose intravenous immunoglobulin. Attenuation of acute, complement-dependent immune damage in a guinea pig model. J Clin Invest 1989;84:1974-81.

10. Anderson, CL. Isolation of the receptor for IgG from a human monocyte cell line (U-937) and from human peripheral blood monocytes. J Exp Med 1982;156:1794-806.

11. Anderson CL, Spence JM, Edward TS, Nusbacher J. Characterization of a polyvalent antibody directed against the IgG Fc receptor of human mononuclear phagocytes. J Immunol 1985;134:465-70.

12. Rossman MD, Chien P, Cassizzi-Cprek A, et al. The binding of monomeric IgG to human blood monocytes and alveolar macrophages. Am Rev Respir Dis 1986;133:292-7.

13. Kurlander RJ, Batker J. The binding of human immunoglobulin G1 monomer and small, covalently cross-linked polymers of immunoglobulin Gl to human peripheral blood monocytes and polymorphonuclear leukocytes. J Clin Invest 1982;69:1-8.

14. Fries LF, Brickman CM, Frank MM. Monocyte receptors for the Fc portion of IgG increase in number in autoimmune hemolytic anemia and other hemolytic states are decreased by glucocorticoid therapy. J Immunol 1983;131:1240-5.

15. Anderson CL, Abraham GN. Characterization of the Fc receptor for IgG on a human macrophage cell line, U937. J Immunol 1980; 125:2735-41.

16. Chien P, Pixley A, Stumpo LG, et al. Modulation of the human monocyte binding site for monomeric immunoglobulin G by activated Hageman factor. J Clin Invest 1988;82:1554-9.

17. Schreiber AD, Chien P, Tomaski A, Cines DB. Effect of danazol in immune thrombocytopenic purpura. N Engl J Med 1987;316:503-8.

18. Huber H, Fudenberg HH. The interaction of monocytes and macrophages with immunoglobulins and complement. Ser Haematol 1970; 3:160-75.

19. Huber H, Douglas SD, Nusbacher J, et al. IgG subclass specificity of human monocyte receptor sites. Nature 1971;229:419-20.

20. Allen JM, Seed B. Isolation and expression of functional high-affinity Fc receptor complementary DNAs. Science 1989;243:378-81.

21. Kurlander RJ, Haney AF, Gartrell J. Human peritoneal macrophages possess two populations of IgG Fc receptors. Cell Immunol 1984; 86:479-90.

22. Lubeck MD, Steplewski Z, Baglia F, et al. The interaction of murine IgG subclass proteins with human monocyte Fc receptors. J Immunol 1985;135:1299-304.

23. Anderson GI, Guyre PM, Shitin JC. Monoclonal antibodies to Fc receptors for IgG on human mononuclear phagocytes. Antibody characterization and induction of superoxide production in a monocyte cell line. J Biol Chem 1986;261:12856-64.
24. Frey J, Engelhardt W. Characterization and structural analysis of Fcγ receptors of human monocytes, a monoblast cell line (U937) and a myeloblast cell line (HL-60) by a monoclonal antibody. Eur J Immunol 1987;17:583-91.
25. Dougherty GJ, Selvendran Y, Murdoch S, et al. The human mononuclear phagocyte high affinity Fc receptor, FcRI, defined by a monoclonal antibody, 10.1. Eur J Immunol 1987;17:1453-9.
26. Rossman MD, Chen E, Chien P, Schreiber AD. Modulation of Fcγ receptors on the human macrophage cell line U-937. Cell Immunol 1989;120:174-87.
27. Schreiber AD, Parsons J, McDermott P, Cooper RA. Effect of corticosteroids on the human monocyte receptors for IgG and complement. J Clin Invest 1975;56:1189-97.
28. Comber PG, Gomez F, Rossman MD, Schreiber AD. Receptors for the Fc portion of immunoglobulin G (FcγR) on human monocytes and macrophages. Prog Clin Biol Res 1989;297:273-85.
29. Comber PG, Rossman MD, Rappaport EF, et al. Modulation of human mononuclear phagocyte Fc receptors by glucocorticoids and interferon-γ. Cell Immunol 1989;124:292-307.
30. Guyre PM, Morganelli PM, Miller R. Recombinant immune interferon increases immunoglobulin G Fc receptors on cultured human mononuclear phagocytes. J Clin Invest 1983;72:393-7.
31. Akiyama Y, Lubeck MD, Steplewsky A, Koprowski H. Induction of mouse IgG2a and IgG3 dependent cellular cytotoxicity in the human monocytic cells (U937) by immune interferon. Cancer Res 1984;44:5127-31.
32. Perussia B, Dayton ET, Lazarus R, et al. Immune interferon induces the receptor for monomeric IgG1 on human monocyte and myeloid cells. J Exp Med 1983;158:1092-1113.
33. Girard MT, Hjaltadottir S, Fejes-Toth AN, Guyre PM. Glucocorticoids enhance the gamma-interferon augmentation of human monocyte immunoglobulin G Fc receptor expression. J Immunol 1987;138:3235-41.
34. Rosenfeld SI, Looney RJ, Leddy JP, et al. Human platelet Fc receptor for immunoglobulin G. Identification of 40,000-molecular weight membrane protein shared by monocytes. J Clin Invest 1985;76:2317-22.
35. Liesveld JC, Abboud CN, Looney JR, et al. Expression of IgG Fc receptors in myeloid leukemic cell lines. J Immunol 1988;140:1527-33.
36. Jones DHK, Looney RJ, Anderson CL. Two distinct classes of IgG Fc receptors on a human monocyte line (U937) defined by differences

in binding of murine IgG subclasses at low ionic strength. J Immunol 1985;135:3348-53.

37. King M, McDermott P, Schreiber AD. Characterization of the Fcγ receptor on human platelets. Cell Immunol 1990;128:262-479.

38. Rossman MD, Chen E, Chien P, et al. Fc receptor recognition of IgG ligand by human monocytes and macrophages. Am J Resp Cell Mol Biol 1989;1:211-20.

39. Jungi TW, Lerch PG, Cachelin AB, Morrell A. Monomeric and dimeric IgG1 as probes for assessing high affinity and low affinity receptors for IgG on human monocyte; derived macrophages and on activated macrophages. Mol Immunol 1988;25:719-9.

40. Gomez FP, Chien P, King M, et al. Monocyte Fc receptor recognition of cell bound and aggregated IgG. Blood 1989;74:1058-65.

41. Anderson CL, Ryan DH, Looney RJ, Leary PC. Structural polymorphism of the human monocyte 40 kilodalton Fc receptor for IgG. J Immunol 1987;138:2254-56.

42. Tax WJ, Hermes FF, Willems RW, et al. Fc receptors for mouse IgG1 on human monocytes: Polymorphism and role in antibody-induced T cell proliferation. J Immunol 1984;133:1185-89.

43. Stewart SG, Trounstine ML, Vaux DJT, et al. Isolation and expression of cDNA clones encoding a human receptor for IgG (FcγRII). J Exp Med 1987;166:1668-84.

44. Hibbs ML, Bonadonna L, Scott BM, et al. Molecular cloning of a human immunoglobulin G Fc receptor. Proc Natl Acad Sci USA 1988; 85:2240-4.

45. Stengelin S, Stamenkovic I, Seed B. Isolation of two distinct human Fc receptors by ligand affinity cloning. The Embo J 1988;7:1053-9.

46. Rappaport EF, Cassel DL, McKenzie SE, et al. Expression of FcγRII in hematopoietic cells: Analysis of transcripts encoding the soluble and membrane-associated molecular forms (abstract). Clin Res 1991; 39:151a.

47. Fanger MW, Shen L, Granziana RF, Guyre PM. Cytotoxicity mediated by human Fc receptors for IgG. Immunol Today 1989;10:92-9.

48. Macintyre EA, Roberts PJ, Abdul-Gaffar R, et al. Mechanism of human monocyte activation via the 40-kDa Fc receptor for IgG. J Immunol 1988;141:4333-43.

49. Fleit HB, Wright SD, Unkeless JC. Human neutrophile Fc receptor distribution and structure. Proc Natl Acad Sci USA 1982;79:3275-9.

50. Clarkson SB, Ory PA. CD 16: Developmental regulated IgG Fc receptors on cultured monocytes. J Exp Med 1988;167:408-17.

51. Baumgartner I, Scheiner O, Holzinger C, et al. Expression of VEPJ3 antigen (CDJ6) on native human alveolar macrophages and cultured blood monocytes. Immunobiology 1988;177:317-26.

52. Werner G, von dem Borne AEG Kr, Fos ME, et al. Localization of the human NA1 alloantigen on neutrophil Fc-γ receptors. In: Leukocyte typing II, Vol. 3. Human myeloid and hematopoietic cells. Reinherz

EL, Haynes BF, Nadler LM, Bernstein ID, eds. Oxford: Oxford University Press, 1986:109-21.

53. Tetteroo PAT, van der Schoot CE, Visser FJ, Bos MJE, von dem Borne AEG Kr. Three different types of Fcγ receptors on human leucocytes defined by workshop antibodies: FcγRI$_{low}$ of neutrophils, Fcγr$_{low}$ of K/NK lymphocytes, and FcγRII. In: McMichael A, ed. Leucocyte typing III: white cell differentiation antigens. Oxford: Oxford University Press, 1987:702-6.

54. Huizinga TWJ, van der Schoot CE, Jost C, et al. The PI-linked receptor FcRIII is released on stimulation of neutrophils. Nature 1988;333:667-9.

55. Simmons D, Seed B. The Fcγ receptor of natural killer cells is a phospholipid-linked membrane protein (published erratum appears in Nature 1989;340:662). Nature 1988;333:568-70.

56. Darby C, Chien P, Rossman MD, Schreiber AD. Monocyte/macrophage FcγRIII, unlike FcγRIII on neutrophils, is not PI-linked protein. Blood 1990;75:2396-400.

57. Clarkson SB, Bussel JB, Kimberly RP, et al. Treatment of refractory immune thrombocytopenic purpura with an anti-Fcγ gamma-receptor antibody. N Engl J Med 1986;314:1236-9.

58. Schreiber AD, Gomez F, Levinson AI, Rossman MD. The Fcγ receptors on human macrophages. Transf Med Rev. 1989;3:281-93.

59. Sultan Y, Kazatchkine MD, Maisonneuve P, Nydegger UE. Anti-idiotypic suppression of autoantibodies to Factor VIII (antihaemophilic factor) by high dose intravenous gammaglobulin. Lancet 1984;2:765-8.

In: Sacher RA, Brubaker DB, Kasprisin DO and McCarthy LJ, eds.
Cellular and Humoral Immunotherapy and Apheresis
Arlington, VA: American Association of Blood Banks, 1991

2

Hemapheresis vs Intravenous Immune Globulin

Duke O. Kasprisin, MD, and Kenneth C. Hoffman, MD

THE RECENT GROWTH OF hemapheresis has been noticeably limited to the treatment of autoimmune diseases. In an American Association of Blood Banks (AABB) survey of hemapheresis usage from 1982-1985, the reported usage of plasma exchange in the treatment of Guillain-Barré syndrome increased by 385% and treatment of myasthenia gravis increased by 327%.[1] Most of this increase was due to a larger number of centers submitting reports of their activity from 1982-1985. However, these two diseases accounted for a larger percentage of the total cases. Guillain-Barré syndrome increased from 16% of all plasma exchange procedures in 1982 to 22% by 1985. This increase was probably due to the strength of the data presented by the Guillain-Barré Syndrome Study Group.[2]

Intravenous gammaglobulin (IVIgG) initially was licensed for the treatment of primary immunodeficiency, eg, common variable immunodeficiency, severe combined immunodeficiency and primary immunoglobulin deficiency. Its use has been expanded to treatment of preterm infants, patients with secondary immunodeficiencies [eg, AIDS, chronic lymphocytic leukemia (CLL)] and patients with autoimmune diseases [ie, idiopathic thrombocytopenic purpura (ITP)]. With the success of IVIgG in the treatment of ITP, additional trials were undertaken to see if this therapy would be useful in the treatment of other autoimmune diseases. This chapter will examine the data concerning the treatment of autoimmune diseases by plasma exchange and IVIgG. Since both have been used to treat

---

Duke O. Kasprisin, MD, Chief Medical Officer, American Red Cross Blood Services—Oklahoma Region, and Associate Clinical Professor, University of Oklahoma Health Sciences Center, Tulsa Medical College; and Kenneth C. Hoffman, MD, Medical Director, American Red Cross Blood Services—Oklahoma Region, Clinical Assistant Professor, University of Oklahoma Health Sciences Center, Tulsa Medical College and Chief of Blood Bank, St. John Medical Center, Tulsa, Oklahoma

some of the same autoimmune diseases, controlled trials should be conducted to decide which therapy is better or whether a combination of both will prove superior to either one separately.

Mechanisms of Action for Intravenous Gammaglobulin

IVIgG appears to work via multiple mechanisms that may act individually or in combination. Five major mechanisms of action have been proposed to account for the manner in which IVIgG works in ITP (blockage of phagocytic cell Fc receptors, interference with the binding of antiplatelet antibody, decreased production of antiplatelet antibody, increased production of platelets, resolution of a viral infection). In utilizing IVIgG for treating thrombocytopenia two mechanisms are probable, ie, blockage of the mononuclear phagocytic system Fc receptors by the gammaglobulin and interference with the binding of the antiplatelet antibody. Fehr et al[3] as well as Bussel and coworkers[4] have shown prolongation of the time it takes to clear antibody-coated red cells from the circulation following IVIgG infusions. It was suggested that antibody-coated platelets had a similarly prolonged survival. The blockage of free Fc receptors is probably due to competition from the increased numbers of monomeric IVIgG molecules. The dramatic increase in platelet count following infusion of IVIgG tends to confirm Fc receptor blockage as a mechanism. Decreased antiplatelet antibody synthesis has been considered a long-term effect, but the evidence in support of this is not apparent. The possibility of stimulation of a suppressor cell by the IVIgG, thus establishing a lower level of antiplatelet antibody, requires more investigation. In thrombocytopenia the possible effect of increasing peripheral platelet counts may be in part due to the enhancement of platelet production since a mononuclear phagocytic system blockage in the marrow would decrease the crossreaction of antibodies with megakaryocytes. An additional possibility may be the resolution of persistent viral infection by the IVIgG that may have been the original cause of the disease.[4]

The mechanisms by which IVIgG may alter the course of diseases such as Guillain-Barré syndrome, myasthenia gravis and thrombotic thrombocytopenic purpura are theoretical and require more study before conclusions can be drawn. In diseases where an autoantibody or immune complex is responsible for disease, it has been proposed that IVIgG is effective by blockage of Fc receptors or immunosuppression by alteration of the reticuloendothelial (RE) system, T-cell subsets or B-cell function, both spontaneous and mitogen-stimulated.[5] Another unproven mechanism is the reaction of anti-idiotypic antibodies present in IVIgG preparations with epitopes on autoantibodies or immune complexes.[6] More needs to be understood about the basic disease processes before the beneficial effects of IVIgG therapy can be explained.

Minnefor and Oleske[7] proposed a more simplistic mechanism for the effectiveness of IVIgG. They believe the elevation in gammmaglobulin level could allow this protein to function more effectively. In addition, the correction of any imbalances in IgG subclasses, whether congenital or acquired, could explain favorable responses especially in those disorders where persistent infection causes production of an autoantibody or immune complex. Fateh-Moghadam et al[8] utilized IVIgG in four cases of myasthenia gravis. They demonstrated that after treatment the anti-acetylcholine receptor antibody levels fell while the total gammaglobulin and total protein levels increased. Their proposed mechanism of action was one of immunosuppression due to either diminished antibody synthesis or increased catabolism. While all of these mechanisms are possible, additional research is necessary to explain the role each plays in the treatment of particular autoimmune diseases.

Mechanism of Therapeutic Apheresis

In most disorders where hemapheresis is indicated, it is assumed that the benefit is accomplished by the removal of an offending agent such as an antibody, an antigen or immune complexes.[9,10] The toxic agent can also be a metabolite as in Refsum's disease. Removal of a nonspecific inflammatory mediator such as complement, C-reactive protein or fibrinogen may also play a role.[10] In a review of hemapheresis, McCullough[11] suggests that removal of excess antibody or antigen may alter the composition of the immune complex and, therefore, change its biologic role. In those diseases where blockage of the RE system is involved in the pathophysiology, hemapheresis may remove immune complexes and allow the unblocked RE system to be more efficient.

When plasma rather than albumin and saline is used as replacement fluid, the plasma may supply some deficient substance or add a regulatory inhibitor or some previously unrecognized "missing" factor. This missing factor could be a gammaglobulin and, therefore, hemapheresis and IVIgG may act in similar fashion. In many diseases the causative agent removed or replaced by hemapheresis is unknown, making it difficult to compare the two therapies. There is little doubt that many other proteins, ions, hormones or materials are removed during hemapheresis and are not replaced by albumin. When an undesirable circulating substance is identified, the utilization of a membrane specifically designed to remove this substance will be an improvement over the simple removal and replacement of plasma.

Indications for Hemapheresis

Several consensus reports have been published concerning the indications for hemapheresis.[12-14] The most recent guidelines were developed by the AABB Extracorporeal Therapy Committee in 1989.[15] Five categories of efficacy were created:

1. Category I—Standard and acceptable under certain circumstances, including primary therapy.
2. Category II—Sufficient evidence to suggest efficacy; acceptable therapy on an adjunctive basis.
3. Category III—Insufficient evidence for efficacy; uncertain benefit/risk ratio. Conditions in this category might be an exceptional effort for an individual case or a research project for numerous cases.
4. Category IV—Lack of efficacy in controlled trials.
5. Category V—Pending further committee investigation.

More complete definitions of these categories and disorders are listed in Tables 2-1 and 2-2. Categories I and II constitute the most widely accepted application of hemapheresis and include several autoimmune diseases that could be candidates for IVIgG as an alternate therapy.

The only autoimmune disease for which IVIgG is licensed is ITP, a Category III condition. Since the success of hemapheresis in the treatment of ITP has been limited, it is unlikely that there will be controlled trials to compare hemapheresis to IVIgG treatment. However, there are ongoing trials and/or anecdotal reports of improvement with IVIgG for common ailments in Categories I and II.

Clinical Comparisons of Intravenous Gammaglobulin and Hemapheresis

ITP was the first autoimmune disease to be successfully treated with IVIgG. Several preparations are now licensed for this purpose. Clinical trials showing the efficacy of IVIgG in the treatment of ITP and its possible mechanisms of action have been reviewed recently. Since most pediatric patients with acute ITP recover spontaneously without treatment, the role for IVIgG is limited to those children at high risk of intracranial hemorrhage. It is difficult to determine which subgroups of these patients are most likely to be at risk. However, platelet counts $<100 \times 10^9$/L ($<100,000$ μL) and clinical hemorrhage, hematuria, hematochezia or continually developing petechiae and purpura may indicate that a patient is a candidate for this therapy.[4]

Adults with acute ITP are less likely to improve spontaneously and, therefore, may undergo splenectomy more often and may have other conditions (eg, diabetes mellitus, osteoporosis, ulcers or immunodeficiencies) that prevent steroid treatment. IVIgG can produce long-term

Table 2-1. Guidelines for Therapeutic Hemapheresis— Category Definitions

CATEGORY I

Conditions for which therapeutic hemapheresis is standard and acceptable under certain circumstances. Included in this category are those diseases for which therapeutic hemapheresis is considered to be first-line therapy, or a valuable adjunct to other initial therapies, under the appropriate clinical circumstances. This does not imply that hemapheresis is mandatory, but rather that it plays a standard and acceptable role in treatment. Evidence of efficacy in this category is derived from controlled or well-designed clinical trials, or from a broad base of published experience.

CATEGORY II

Most of the diseases in this category have been studied sufficiently that the efficacy of plasma exchange treatment is generally accepted. However, plasma exchange therapy is considered as an adjunct to other available treatment modalities, and is not approved as a treatment by itself. A few prospective randomized controlled studies have been performed for some of these diseases, but often they are lacking, and only case studies and reports of small numbers of patients are available.

CATEGORY III

There is insufficient evidence to evaluate efficacy. There is an uncertain benefit to risk ratio. This category includes those diseases for which there are numerous anecdotal reports without an adequate consensus to conclude whether hemapheresis is beneficial. Also included in this category are those diseases in which there are trials with conflicting results, or those diseases where too few case reports utilizing hemapheresis permit evaluation. The use of hemapheresis in these conditions might be an exceptional effort for an individual case where other conventional therapies have failed. It may also be used for numerous cases under a research protocol with Institutional Review Board approval.

CATEGORY IV

Controlled trials, if available, have shown no therapeutic efficacy. Anecdotal and uncontrolled studies do not demonstrate beneficial effect. Plasma exchange for these diseases is discouraged and should be done only with an approved research protocol.

CATEGORY V

Pending further investigation by Committee.

Table 2-2. Guidelines for Therapeutic Hemapheresis—Diseases

CATEGORY I

Standard and acceptable under certain circumstances, including primary therapy.

PLASMA EXCHANGE
Coagulation factor inhibitors
Cryoglobulinemia
Goodpasture's syndrome
Guillain-Barré syndrome
Homozygous familial hypercholesterolemia
Hyperviscosity syndrome
Myasthenia gravis
Posttransfusion purpura
Refsum's disease
Thrombotic thrombocytopenic purpura

CYTAPHERESIS
Leukemia with hyperleukocytosis syndromes
Sickle cell syndromes (also see Category IV)
Thrombocytosis *symptomatic*

CATEGORY II

Sufficient evidence to suggest efficacy; acceptable therapy on an adjunctive basis.

PLASMA EXCHANGE
Chronic inflammatory demyelinating polyneuropathy
Cold agglutinin disease
Drug overdose and poisoning (involving protein-bound toxins)
Hemolytic uremic syndrome
Idiopathic thrombocytopenic purpura (ITP) (Protein A chromatography)
Pemphigus vulgaris
Rapidly progressive glomerulonephritis (RPGN)
Systemic vasculitis (primary, or in association with SLE and RA)

CYTAPHERESIS
Cutaneous T-cell lymphoma
Hairy cell leukemia
Rheumatoid arthritis

CATEGORY III

Insufficient evidence for efficacy; uncertain benefit/risk ratio. Conditions that may fall into this category might be an exceptional effort for an individual case or a research project for numerous cases.

PLASMA EXCHANGE
Allo-antibody removal (red cell, platelets, HLA)
Maternal treatment of maternal fetal incompatibility (hemolytic disease of the newborn)
Hyperthyroidism, including thyroid storm
Multiple sclerosis
Polymyositis/dermatomyositis
Progressive systemic sclerosis
Pure red cell aplasia
Warm autoimmune hemolytic anemia

CYTAPHERESIS
Multiple sclerosis
Renal transplant rejection

There are numerous other diseases for which plasmapheresis has been done from which no conclusions can be drawn.

CATEGORY IV

Lack of efficacy in controlled trials.

PLASMA EXCHANGE
AIDS (for symptoms of immunodeficiency)
Amyotrophic lateral sclerosis
Aplastic anemia
Fulminant hepatic failure
Psoriasis
Renal transplant rejection
Rheumatoid arthritis
Schizophrenia

benefit and can be used to postpone or avoid splenectomy or prepare patients for surgery.[16]

IVIgG has also been shown to be beneficial in chronic ITP in children. Complete remission can occur with IVIgG alone but the majority of patients with very low platelet counts can be stabilized with or without continued infusion without resorting to splenectomy. As many as 65% of these patients could avoid splenectomy with IVIgG.[17-20]

In adult chronic ITP, 5-10% of splenectomized patients will continue to have dangerously low platelet counts. Many of these patients can be helped, at least in the short term, with IVIgG. Studies have found 70-80% have at least a short-term improvement and in one study 12 of 30 who received it as maintenance therapy improved enough to stabilize without further therapy.[4]

Using plasma exchange in ITP is now rare since the advent of IVIgG and comparative studies seem unlikely. There is limited experience using the two therapies together in the treatment of complex cases.

Plasma exchange has become an accepted therapy for thrombotic thrombocytopenic purpura (TTP) and posttransfusion purpura (PTP). These conditions are extremely uncommon and acceptance of plasma exchange in their treatment was by consensus rather than controlled clinical trials. Occasional reports of successful response has been associated with IVIgG in the treatment of TTP, but most of these patients received multiple therapies including plasma exchange; thus, the value of IVIgG is difficult to evaluate.[21-24] The authors have not had any success using IVIgG in patients refractory to plasma exchange, steroids and other therapies. PTP is rare and experience with IVIgG is too limited for conclusions, although a theoretical rationale exists for trying IVIgG in this disorder.[7]

Guillain-Barré syndrome and myasthenia gravis are the two disorders most commonly treated with plasma exchange. Both ailments have also been treated with IVIgG. The value of plasma exchange has been proven in a well-controlled randomized study. To evaluate whether IVIgG is comparable therapy, a randomized multicenter trial of IVIgG vs plasma exchange has been established. Preliminary results indicate that there may be improved functional recovery for patients receiving IVIgG but the study is not yet completed.[5]

Anecdotal reports about the use of IVIgG in the treatment of myasthenia gravis have been very promising.[7,8,25] Although the numbers treated are very small, most patients appeared to respond when treated with IVIgG alone. Further study is warranted based on these preliminary results.

Other diseases occasionally treated by plasma exchange that have been reported to have been treated by IVIgG include autoimmune hemolytic anemia[26] and Rh maternal-fetal incompatibility.[27,28] Chronic inflammatory demyelinating polyneuropathy has been successfully treated with IVIgG in several small studies.[5]

Other Comparisons Between Intravenous Gammaglobulin and Hemapheresis

Risks

To compare the efficacy of hemapheresis vs IVIgG in treating autoimmune diseases, the risks of each must be balanced against the benefits. Neither modality is free of complications but the frequency of problems can be affected by the manner in which it is administered.

The indications and adverse reaction rate of IVIgG depend on the method of manufacture. All preparations are licensed for patients with primary immunodeficiency but only some are licensed for ITP and the prevention of bacterial infections in CLL. In general, the reaction rate is 1-15% for primary immunodeficiency states and less for ITP.[5] It is assumed that the rate of reaction for autoimmune diseases would be similar to ITP. Specific problems associated with each preparation are provided in the package insert. The most severe complications of IVIgG are immediate anaphylactoid and hypersensitivity reactions due to prior sensitization to certain antigens, most commonly IgA. Some hypo- and agammaglobulinemic patients are IgA deficient and some of these patients develop anti-IgA antibodies. If IVIgG therapy becomes necessary, these patients must be treated with an IgA-depleted IVIgG preparation.

Other adverse reactions to IVIgG include chills, fever, nausea, vomiting, flushing, dizziness, diaphoresis, chest tightness and hypotension. Reactions can frequently be diminished by slowing the rate of infusion. Headaches appear to be more common in ITP patients receiving high doses of IVIgG. The causes of these reactions are unknown.

Complications of hemapheresis have been reviewed recently by Westphal.[29] Adverse reactions accompanying blood or hemapheresis donation can also occur in therapeutic hemapheresis patients. Hematomas, syncope, hypovolemia, hypervolemia, chills, citrate toxicity, air embolism, allergic reactions and complement activation have been reported. Hemapheresis procedures can also exaggerate clinical problems in critically ill patients. Complications due to machine and plasticware failures are uncommon and have been described in detail by Westphal.[29]

The frequency and severity of adverse reactions depend, in part, on the replacement fluid used during the procedure. When blood and blood components are used as replacement, there is the risk of transmitting hepatitis, human immunodeficiency virus and other transfusion-transmitted infections. Fresh frozen plasma (FFP) is routinely used as a replacement fluid with certain diseases, eg, TTP. FFP is associated with numerous problems. In addition to the risk of transfusion-transmitted infections, allergic and febrile reactions occur approximately once in 720 infusions.[30] FFP also contains higher concentrations of citrate than other replacement fluids.

Plasma protein fraction has caused hypotension when it is rapidly administered as is the case in hemapheresis. Plasma protein fraction and albumin are iso-osmotic to plasma and are manufactured in a fashion that removes the risk of viral transmission. Plasma protein fraction, albumin and crystalloids do not replace the clotting factors, immunoglobulins and other substances present in FFP. The removal of these substances during plasma exchange rarely causes problems because of their rapid equilibration.

In a study of pediatric patients receiving plasma exchange with saline and albumin replacement, the prothrombin time and partial thromboplastin time were elevated and the individual clotting factors, high-molecular-weight kininogen, prekallikrein, antithrombin III and plasminogen were reduced but returned to normal 24 hours after the procedure. No bleeding occurred.[31]

In adults undergoing hemapheresis, hemorrhagic complications were also uncommon.[32] Immunoglobulins are also effectively removed by plasma exchange but infections are rare. However, infection has been associated with the removal of immunoglobulins in the treatment of rapidly progressive crescentic glomerulonephritis.[33] Replacing immunoglobulins following plasma exchange has been advocated by some but is seldom used.

Huestis[34] recently reported 59 deaths associated with hemapheresis worldwide. Of the 45 cases evaluated, the most common causes of death were cardiovascular and respiratory problems. Other causes included anaphylaxis, pulmonary thromboembolism, vascular perforation, hepatitis, hemorrhage and sepsis. In those cases where the replacement fluids were identified, 25 of 42 received FFP. This is significant considering that FFP is uncommonly used as a replacement fluid. This is particularly worrisome since one of the mechanisms by which plasma exchange may work is by replacing a missing factor supplied by the FFP, as in TTP. If the mechanism of action of plasma exchange is due to a regulatory effect by the immunoglobulins in FFP, IVIgG replacement would be safer.

Costs

It is difficult to compare the costs of treatment by IVIgG or hemapheresis. The number of procedures, type of replacement fluids, dose and schedule of IVIgG must all be taken into account to evaluate which therapy is most costly. In TTP, IVIgG will most likely be used as an adjunct to plasma exchange and no comparison exists between the two therapies. Plasma exchange will probably be continued after IVIgG is started, and it will be impossible to estimate if the addition of the IVIgG shortens the disease process. Large doses of IVIgG, as are used in ITP, are usually more expensive than a single hemapheresis procedure, depending on which replacement fluids are used. However, new shorter dosage regimens of

IVIgG, eg, 2 days of 400 mg/kg/day may be less expensive than longer treatment schedules by hemapheresis. Some comparison can be made in treating Guillain-Barré syndrome for 5 days using albumin and saline as replacement for the plasma removed by hemapheresis or using 400 mg/kg/day of IVIgG. If the patient required hemapheresis for more than 5 days but the IVIgG was effective within 5 days, the decrease in therapy as well as in hospitalization would more than offset the additional costs of the IVIgG. Realistically, however, one must individualize each case and this can only be done retrospectively. Many other factors must be considered in cost comparisons such as the use of ventilators, numerous blood gas or electrolyte determinations, and the degree of nursing care in an intensive care unit.

Other Considerations

Further controlled trials will be necessary to compare the effectiveness of IVIgG vs hemapheresis. Since the mechanism of action for both therapies is poorly understood, it is difficult to hypothesize which modality will be beneficial without trials. Numerous difficulties will occur during these trials. It is unknown whether the various preparations of IVIgG are equivalent. Failure of one preparation does not necessarily imply that IVIgG in general is of little value. The manner in which hemapheresis is conducted, its frequency, type and amount of replacement fluids, amount of plasma exchanged and many other factors have not been quantified and comparison to IVIgG will be difficult. Since plasma exchange with plasma replacement may be beneficial in some disease due to immunoglobulins in the plasma, the additional comparison of plasma exchange with IVIgG replacement may need to be added to the clinical trials of IVIgG and hemapheresis.

References

1. Taft EG. Trends in hemapheresis experience. In: Westphal RG, Kasprisin DO, eds. Current status of hemapheresis: Indications, technology and complications. Arlington, VA: American Association of Blood Banks, 1987:1-7.
2. Guillain-Barré Study Group. Plasmapheresis and acute Guillain-Barré syndrome. Neurology 1985;35:1096-104.
3. Fehr J, Hofmann V, Kappeler U. Transient reversal of thrombocytopenia in idiopathic thrombocytopenic purpura by high-dose intravenous gammaglobulin. N Engl J Med 1982;62:480-6.
4. Bussel JB. Intravenous immunoglobulin therapy of immune hematological disease. In: Garner RJ, Sacher RA, eds. Intravenous

gammaglobulin therapy. Arlington, VA: American Association of Blood Banks, 1988:99-112.

5. NIH Consensus Conference. Intravenous immunoglobulin. Prevention and treatment of disease. JAMA 1990;264:3189-93.

6. Berchtold P, Dale GL, Tani P, McMillan R. Inhibition of autoantibody binding to platelet glycoprotein IIb/IIIa by anti-idiotypic antibodies in intravenous gammaglobulin. Blood 1989;74:2414-17.

7. Minnefor AB, Oleske JM. IV immune globulin: Efficacy and safety. Hosp Pract 1987;22(10):171-86.

8. Fateh-Moghadam A, Besinger U, Guersen RG. High-dose intravenous gammaglobulin for myasthenia gravis. Lancet 1984;1:848-9.

9. Schumak KH, Rock GA. Therapeutic plasma exchange. N Engl J Med 1984;310(12):762-71.

10. Singsen BH. Plasmapheresis: A pediatric perspective. J Pediatr 1981; 98:232-4.

11. McCullough J, Chopek M. Therapeutic plasma exchange. Lab Med 1981;12:745-53.

12. Report of the AMA Panel on Therapeutic Plasmapheresis. Current status of therapeutic plasmapheresis and related technique. JAMA 1985;253:819-25.

13. Klein HG, Balow JE, Dau PC, et al. Clinical applications of therapeutic apheresis. Report of the Clinical Applications Committee, American Society for Apheresis. J Clin Apheresis 1986;3(1),1-92.

14. Consensus Conference. The utility of therapeutic plasmapheresis for neurological disorders. JAMA 1986;256:1333-37.

15. AABB Extracorporeal Therapy Committee. Guidelines for therapeutic hemapheresis. Arlington, VA: American Association of Blood Banks, 1989.

16. Newland AC, Treleaven JG, Minchinton RM. High-dose intravenous IgG in adults with autoimmune thrombocytopenia. Lancet 1983; 1:84-7.

17. Bussel JB, Shulman I, Hilgartner MW, et al. Intravenous use of gammaglobulin in the treatment of chronic immune thrombocytopenic purpura as a means to defer splenectomy. J Pediatr 1983; 103:651-4.

18. Hollenberg JP, Subak LL, Ferry JJ, Bussel JB. Cost-effectiveness of splenectomy versus intravenous gammaglobulin in treatment of chronic immune thrombocytopenic purpura in childhood. J Pediatr 1988; 112:530-9.

19. Warrier AL, Lusher JM. Intravenous gammaglobulin treatment of chronic idiopathic thrombocytopenic purpura in children. Am J Med 1984;76:193-8.

20. Imholz B, Imbach P, Baumgartner C, et al. Intravenous immunoglobulin (IVIgG) for previously treated acute or for chronic idiopathic thrombocytopenic purpura (ITP) in childhood: A prospective multicenter study. Blut 1988;56:63-8.

21. Finn NG, Wang JC, Hong KJ. High-dose intravenous gamma-immu-noglobulin infusion in the treatment of thrombotic thrombocytope-nic purpura. Arch Intern Med 1987;147:2165-7.
22. Viero P, Cortelazzo S, Buelli M, et al. Thrombotic thrombocytopenic purpura and high-dose immunoglobulin treatment. Ann Intern Med 1986;104:282.
23. Messmore HL, Teshwant C, Remlineer K, et al. Intravenous gamma globulin in refractory thrombotic thrombocytopenic purpura. Thromb Haemost 1985;54:127.
24. Gilcher RO. Refractory TTP responding to I.V. gamma globulin (ab-stract). Blood 1985;64:(Suppl):1237a.
25. Gajdos PH, Outin H, Elkharrat D, et al. High-dose intravenous gam-maglobulin for myasthenia gravis. Lancet 1984;1:406-7.
26. Bussel A, Jaisson F, Janvier M, et al. Utilisation des gammaglobulines intraveineuses à fortes doses dans le traîtement des anémies hémo-lytiques auto-immunes. Nouv Presse Med 1983;12:41.
27. Berlin G, Selbing A, Ryden G. Rhesus haemolytic disease treated with high-dose intravenous immunoglobulin. Lancet 1985;1:1153.
28. de la Cámara C, Arrieta R, González A, et al. High-dose intravenous immunoglobulin as the sole prenatal treatment for severe Rh immu-nization. N Engl J Med 1988;318:519-20.
29. Westphal RG. Complications of hemapheresis. In: Westphal RG, Kas-prisin DO, eds. Current status of hemapheresis: Indications, technol-ogy and complications. Arlington, VA: American Association of Blood Banks, 1987:87-104.
30. Kasprisin DO, Yogore MG, Salmassi S, Bolf EC. Blood components and transfusion reactions. Plasma Ther Transf Technol 1981;2:25-9.
31. Rao AK, Schneider B, Beckett C, et al. The hemostatic system in children undergoing intensive plasma exchange. J Pediatr 1982; 100:69-75.
32. Keller AJ, Chirnside A, Urbaniak SJ. Coagulation abnormalities pro-duced by plasma exchange on the cell separator with special refer-ence to fibrinogen and platelet levels. Br J Haematol 1979;42:593-603.
33. Wing EJ, Bruns FJ, Fraley DS, et al. Infectious complications with plasmapheresis in rapidly progressive glomerulonephritis. JAMA 1980;244:2423-6.
34. Huestis DW. Complications of therapeutic apheresis. In: Valbonesi M, Pineda AA, Biggs JC, eds. Therapeutic hemapheresis. Milan: Wichtig Editore, 1986:179-86.

In: Sacher RA, Brubaker DB, Kasprisin DO and McCarthy LJ, eds.
Cellular and Humoral Immunotherapy and Apheresis
Arlington, VA: American Association of Blood Banks, 1991

3

Immunoaffinity Apheresis Columns: Clinical Applications and Therapeutic Mechanisms of Action

Alvaro A. Pineda, MD

FOR CENTURIES MEDICAL PRACTITIONERS have entertained the notion of abnormal blood composition as a crucial element of disease. This has resulted in a number of empirical practices directed at eliminating undesirable materials from blood. Bloodletting, a direct and unselective approach, evolved with time as a therapeutic technique used in ancient times and even today. Plasmapheresis, a technique of more recent introduction for the extraction of plasma, is recognized as the precursor of modern donor and therapeutic hemapheresis. The latter, represented mainly by plasma exchange or therapeutic plasmapheresis, gained wide application in the past two decades.

The increased use of plasma exchange, an unselective wholesale removal of plasma, in a variety of disorders provided the impetus for the selective removal of plasma constituents. A recently introduced, more selective removal of plasma constituents can be accomplished by chemical, physical or immunologic means in either off-line or on-line fashion. The plasma constituents are extracted by perfusion of plasma (plasma-perfusion) or whole blood (hemoperfusion) over affinity columns, filters or cartridges containing immobilized sorbents or ligands. These types of perfusion permit replacement with autologous blood components, obviating the use of homologous blood components or products with their risks and costs. Selective extraction is also more physiologic, potentially more economical and as efficient as plasma exchange. This chapter focuses on techniques that use immunologic means to selectively extract plasma constituents by perfusion or extracorporeal treatment.

Alvaro A. Pineda, MD, Professor of Laboratory Medicine and Director, Apheresis Laboratory, Mayo Clinic, Rochester, Minnesota

In this context, we define immunoapheresis as the extraction of immune reactants from the patient's circulation by immunologic means. The definition also includes removal of nonimmunologic substances by immune-mediated processing. The basic technology used to extract materials is affinity chromatography. This technology uses a substance (ligand or sorbent) with a selective binding affinity coupled to an insoluble matrix (carrier) to bind its complementary substance(s) from a mixture of materials in solution or suspension. The sorbent or ligand linked to the carrier (immobilized) can be an antigen or an antibody or an immune reactant, and as such it absorbs its homologous reciprocal or antithetical material. Removal of antigen, antibody or immune complex and other immune reactants is discussed with emphasis on clinical applications and mechanisms of action.

Types of Immunoaffinity Apheresis Columns

The several types of immunoaffinity columns available vary in the sorbent or ligand used, the carrier and the material extracted. Regarding the latter, columns extract antigens, antibodies or immune complexes. A number of carriers have been used; these include Sepharose®, agarose, collodion-charcoal, polyvinyl alcohol gel, polyacrolein microspheres, glass beads and silica. Typically, the carriers are inert substances, highly biocompatible with human plasma and generally incapable of activating systems such as complement, kinins, etc. Generally, they require chemical activation for what is typically a covalent linkage of the sorbent. Despite this strong linkage, there can be leakage of the sorbent.

The ligand or sorbent varies according to the specificity of the material being removed. For instance, a number of sorbents such as concanavalin A, DNA, insulin, heparin and red blood cells have been utilized to create absorption systems used experimentally. Other sorbents have become parts of systems that progressed to human application. They include low density lipoprotein (LDL) antibody and heparin to extract LDL, staphylococcal protein A to extract IgG and immune complexes, synthetic blood group substances to remove isoagglutinins, DNA to remove the corresponding antibody and amino acids to extract immune gammaglobulins (IgG). The initial experience with these systems has been reviewed.[1-2] Some of the systems, however, deserve a brief description because of their more advanced application.

For antibody extraction, there is a system based on hydrophobic chromatography that is selective for proteins, particularly IgG and fibrinogen. The sorbent in the amino acid tryptophan is linked to the carrier polyvinyl alcohol gel. It has exhibited a greater affinity for specific antibodies, such as acetylcholine receptor antibody, than for IgG and other proteins. One of the more extensively applied systems uses an antibody raised in sheep to human apolipoprotein B and linked to Sepharose®. It removes LDL from patients with familial hypercholesterolemia.[3] It is efficient, safe, specific and capable of reducing circulating cholesterol levels by 70% with the extraction of up to 10 grams of LDL.

Alternatives

Filtration technology, widely utilized in hemodialysis and hemofiltration for decades, has recently been introduced in therapeutic hemapheresis.[4] Filtration uses microporous membranes made of a wide variety of materials and assembled in either a parallel plate or flat membrane and hollow fiber. The membranes function as screens, allowing selective passage of materials through pores of varying sizes. The rate of passage is related to the sieving properties of the membrane, transmembrane pressure, membrane area, flow rate and blood characteristics. Membrane filtration is used to separate plasma from the formed elements of blood, producing cell-free plasma. For selective extraction of plasma constituents, a variant of filtration, ultrafiltration, has been applied.

Secondary membrane filtration or cascade filtration is a form of ultrafiltration employed to achieve a greater selectivity in the removal of plasma constituents. With ultrafiltration, the plasma is subfractionated with filters of variable porosity or subjected to low temperatures to induce cyroprecipitation of proteins. Techniques of cryoprecipitation and filtration or ultrafiltration are designed to extract high-molecular-weight components–a fraction containing antibodies and immune complexes with concomitant generation of modified plasma suitable for autologous use. Ultrafiltration systems are available for extraction of pathogenic substances (large molecules), which are retained on the basis of the pore size of the filter. Currently available filters have pores suitable to pass albumin but capable of retaining the larger plasma proteins.

Typically, plasma separated by centrifugation or filtration (primary) is passed through an ultrafilter, generally the hollow fiber type. The resulting filtrate has a higher ratio of albumin to globulin than that of plasma. Thus, the albumin-rich fraction (filtrate) can serve as autologous replacement since it is largely free of pathogenic elements such as immune complexes and antibodies that are retained by the filter.[5] Other pathogenic materials, for instance, low density lipoproteins, can also be excluded on the basis of size. Ultrafiltration is more selective than plasmapheresis but not as specific as immunoadsorption.

Another form of ultrafiltration is the technique of cold ultrafiltration, which is enhanced by cryogelation of high-molecular-weight proteins. In this procedure, plasma separated by filtration is cooled to promote gelation and cryoprecipitation of macromolecule solutes with molecular weight in excess of 100,000 daltons.[6] The cryoprecipitable macromolecular elements of plasma are retained by an in-line ultrafilter. The filtered plasma is subsequently reunited with the formed elements of blood for reinfusion. This system is FDA-approved but has found only very limited application in the treatment of rheumatoid arthritis.

Toxicity

Adverse reactions of varying severity have been observed in humans treated with immunoaffinity apheresis columns. Severe reactions and even fatalities have been documented in patients being treated with staphylococcal protein A columns. In 1983, Young and co-workers reported on the cardiopulmonary toxicity observed in patients with breast carcinoma treated with immobilized protein A.[7] The report defined for the first time the physiologic basis of the cardiopulmonary toxicity in humans as observed by these authors as well as by others who had described the symptomatology consistently observed since the early application of protein A. The authors reported an increased mean blood pressure, systemic vascular resistance, stroke volume, heart rate, cardiac output and rectal temperature occurring within 30 minutes of plasmaperfusion. At 90 minutes, hypotension developed (lowest mean pressure was 59 ± 14 mm Hg) and was associated with a decrease in systemic vascular resistance and total pulmonary resistance.

During the hypotensive episode, values of creatinine clearance and fractional excretion of sodium diminished. Noncardiogenic pulmonary edema appeared occasionally and a single instance of bronchospasm was noted. This toxicity was observed with purified protein A immobilized on collodion charcoal but was similar to hemodynamic toxicity observed with the immobilized heat-killed and formalin-fixed staphylococci. No hemodynamic change occurred when a saline solution was perfused over protein A or when autologous plasma was given without perfusion over the same column. Significant attenuation of the toxicity was observed when modifications of the system were introduced, resulting in reduction of protein A quantity and plasma volumes perfused as well as slowing the plasma perfusion rate. Characterization of the pathophysiologic changes permitted use of a rational pharmacotherapeutic intervention.

Later, Terman and Bertram linked the toxicity and efficacy of the treatment in human malignant disease.[8] Early observations showed that patients responsive to therapy (that is, those who showed antitumor effect) also had systemic side effects of chills, rigor and fever, hypotension and pain localized in the tumor site. Conversely, patients who had lacked adverse effects after treatment with protein A not only failed to show tumoricidal changes but also had tumor progression during therapy. The toxicity they observed was manageable even in severe cases. Hypotension was successfully treated with volume expansion and vasoactive drugs. Fever was attenuated with antipyretics and the rigors were controlled with meperidine (Demerol)® administered intravenously. Bronchospasm was reversed with bronchodilators and corticosteroids.

Products generated after interaction of plasma components (off-line and on-line) with immobilized protein A and those leached from the column in the course of plasma treatments were considered potential etiologic agents that could explain the toxicity. Thus, complement activation and generation of biologically active complement byproducts or leached materials such as protein A and enterotoxins were suspects. A study demonstrated that approximately 5% of commercially purified protein A contained identifiable enterotoxins A and B.[9] Another study documented leakage of protein A in patients treated with plasma perfusion over protein A columns.[10] Complement activation with generation of C3a was also documented and proposed as a possible cause of the reactions.[11] Ample experimental information existed to support the potential causative effect of all or any of the suspected agents, although conclusive proof was lacking.

Protein A produced by several manufacturers is presently made for in-vitro, mostly laboratory use and is not intended to be used as a pharmaceutical. The relative role of protein A in the toxicity remains unknown at this point. In a recent review, Terman discusses the several important biomolecules that either contaminate commercial protein A or are present in plasma that has been perfused over protein A columns.[12] As discussed before, the presence of trace, yet biologically significant amounts of staphylococcal enterotoxins in purified protein A preparations has been confirmed. Likewise, the presence of anaphylotoxins in plasma perfused over protein A has also been confirmed. In addition, conjugates of protein A and IgG with molecular weights ranging from 600,000 to 2,000,000 daltons have been identified in the perfused plasma. These biomolecules are thought to contribute significantly to the toxicity of the column A treatment. Presently, the only FDA-approved protein A affinity column is manufactured by IMRE Corporation (Seattle, WA) under the trade name of Prosorba® column. The column is approved for the treatment of idiopathic thrombocytopenic purpura (ITP). Phase one or toxicity studies demonstrated toxicity in patients with ITP treated with the now commercially approved column.[13] Fourteen different side effects were reported with a predominance of pain, fever, chills and rash affecting from 11% to 26% of patients. The use of the same column in patients with cancer resulted in a 32% rate of reactions in 581 treatments of 60 tumor patients. The reactions were transient, manageable and carried no mortality.[13]

A fatal pulmonary reaction with the Prosorba® column in a patient with pure red cell aplasia has been reported.[14] The patient was severely anemic [hemoglobin = 34 g/L (3.4 g/dL)] and had refused red blood cell transfusion due to religious convictions. The patient received four on-line daily perfusions and reacted during the first procedure with rigors and bronchospasm. For procedures 2, 3 and 4, the patient was heavily premedicated; however, 40 minutes after the fourth procedure was completed, the patient developed dyspnea with bronchospasm, which progressed to a full respiratory arrest and death. The authors concluded that extreme caution must be used when applying the column treatment in patients with poor respiratory reserve.

Clinical Applications

The FDA-licensed protein A column has been utilized to treat patients with ITP (the only clinical application for which the column is currently licensed). A prototype of a protein A column has undergone premarketing trials in this country and has been primarily used to extract circulating antibodies. The FDA-licensed column has also been used to treat mitomycin C associated hemolytic uremic syndrome (HUS) in patients with cancer, mainly breast adenocarcinoma. For the same application, data exist with a homemade protein A column. Finally, the FDA-licensed column has been employed in the treatment of patients with cancer and assessment of safety has been published.[13] Results of the clinical application of the system in the conditions aforementioned follow.

Idiopathic (Immune) Thrombocytopenic Purpura

Idiopathic thrombocytopenic purpura is a primary immune thrombocytopenia that is typically manifested in patients by moderate-to-severe thrombocytopenia, acute bleeding and normal-to-increased megakaryocytes in the bone marrow. Studies strongly suggest that a majority of patients with ITP have an IgG antibody directed against antigens present on the platelet membrane (primarily glycoproteins IIb, IIIa), resulting in sequestration and premature destruction of platelets in the spleen. The mainstay of therapy includes corticosteroids and/or splenectomy, which induce permanent remission in 75% of patients. Refractoriness to established therapy results in a number of patients who are treated with a variety of regimens. Drugs such as IVIG, cyclophosphamide, azathioprine and vincristine have been used in patients failing splenectomy and/or corticosteroids. However, less than 50% of the refractory patients achieve long-term desirable platelet counts.

New therapeutic modalities have been explored to treat patients who fail established therapy. Plasmapheresis has been used with varying degrees of success in uncontrolled series. Although the efficacy of plasmapheresis in adult ITP has not been demonstrated by a controlled study, anecdotal evidence of success has provided enough impetus for the use of a protein A column. An initial study of the Prosorba® column used in 11 patients with immune thrombocytopenia, of whom nine had positive HIV serology, reported an increase in the platelet count of 50% or more in eight patients.[13]   Six of nine patients with positive HIV serology had platelet counts 1.7 to 4.3 times higher than pretreatment counts following four to eight treatments and a decrease of C1q-CIC (immune complex activated complement fragments) to background levels. Those patients judged unresponsive to therapy showed no diminution of platelet-associated IgG or C1q-CIC levels as had those responsive to therapy.

An additional report on the Prosorba® column for the treatment of HIV-associated ITP described results in 29 patients, which included patients reported previously.[15] The mean platelet count of patients before therapy was $52,647 \pm 9,914/\mu L^3$ and none were reported to have bleeding complications. Platelet-associated IgG and CIC (circulating immune complexes) were elevated in all patients. The patients were treated off-line receiving 250 mL of autologous plasma that had been perfused over the column, collected and then reinfused the day of treatment (treatment administered more than one time in all patients). At the completion of four to eight treatments, 16 patients demonstrated a 170-430% increase in their platelet counts with a median duration of response of 8-12 months. Decreased CIC and platelet-associated IgG were noted in all responding patients. Fever and chills were the most frequent toxicity followed by urticaria and musculoskeletal pain. The latter toxicity resembled acute serum sickness and may have been the consequence of a documented activation of the complement cascade.

ITP not related to positive HIV serology has also been treated with the Prosorba® column. Thirteen patients with adult classical ITP were treated with off-line or on-line procedures resulting in three complete remissions [platelet count $>150 \times 10^9/L$ ($>150,000/\mu L$) for 6 or more months], three partial responses [platelet count $50-150 \times 10^9/L$ ($50,000$ to $150,000/\mu L$)] and eight no responses [platelet count $< 50 \times 10^9/L$ ($<50,000/\mu L$)].[16,17] The patients had pretreatment counts of $<50 \times 10^9/L$ ($<50,000/\mu L$) and some had been refractory to conventional therapy. None of the cases was reported to have active bleeding. Nausea, vomiting, headache and fever were the most common adverse effects followed by myalgias, edema and hypotension in order of frequency. In some of the patients responding to therapy, decreased levels of platelet-associated IgG and CIC were documented.

The numbers of patients treated with the Prosorba® column are too small to derive valid conclusions relative to the efficacy of this therapy. There is not yet a published controlled study assessing the efficacy of the column treatment, and it is doubtful one will be available any time soon, since the difficulties of carrying out such a study are formidable and have hindered the study of plasmapheresis and other treatment modalities. None of the reports to date has included treatment of cases of life-threatening severe immune thrombocytopenia consistently unresponsive to conventional therapy. Use of the protein A column clearly is not first-line therapy and needs to be compared scientifically with IVIG and plasmapheresis to determine its efficacy. The toxicity, although manageable in the cases reported, occasionally has been severe and merited discontinuation in two patients. Toxicity appears to be more severe than that reported for IVIG and therapeutic plasmapheresis.

Hemolytic Uremic Syndrome/Thrombotic Thrombocytopenic Purpura

Protein A immunoadsorption has been used to treat patients with cancer chemotherapy-associated thrombotic thrombocytopenic purpura/hemolytic uremic syndrome (CCATTP/HUS). Korec and co-workers first reported 11 patients with cancer who had been treated with mitomycin and who subsequently developed HUS.[18] Significant elevations in platelets and red blood cell counts were observed in nine patients and stabilization of progressive renal impairment was achieved in six patients. Long-term control was achieved in seven patients (median follow-up of 9 months) who were in tumor remission. Three patients with tumor recurrence had an incomplete and short-lived response. Protein A immunoperfusion resulted in complete clearance of pretreatment elevated levels of circulating immune complexes in eight patients. An unpublished report by HW Snyder et al describes the use of the Prosorba® column in 54 patients with CCATTP/HUS treated in 25 US institutions, an average of six times over a 2.5-week period. Improvement in hemolytic anemia, thrombocytopenia and renal function was achieved in 69% of patients and >8 months survival was observed in 42% of evaluable patients. These response rates are significantly greater than historical controls receiving no treatment or receiving conventional therapy including plasmapheresis (HW Snyder, unpublished observation). Of greater importance is the observation that in patients without recurrent tumor, the incidence of improvement in patients with CCATTP/HUS who received protein A column treatment was 96% and the survival of >8 months was 80%. The adverse effects (ie, fever, chills, nausea/vomiting or pain) observed with therapy occurred in 44% of procedures and were generally mild and manageable.

Between 2 and 10% of cancer patients treated with chemotherapeutic drugs, ie, mitomycin C, bleomycin and cis-platin, develop CCATTP/HUS, characterized by thrombocytopenia, progressive renal impairment and microangiopathic hemolytic anemia.[19] The diffuse intraluminal thrombi around endothelial lesions in the microcirculation probably account for hemolysis, microangiopathic erythrocytic changes and renal failure.[20] Circulating immune complexes and high platelet aggregation activity in these patients support an immunologic etiology for the primary endothelial cell injury solely or in combination with injury caused by the chemotherapy. No effective therapy has existed for this condition, which causes significant mortality (50% within 2 months and 75% within 4 months of diagnosis). Therapeutic plasmapheresis is largely unsuccessful (Pineda, unpublished data); in fact 13 patients in Snyder's series (HW Snyder, unpublished observations) had failed to respond to plasmapheresis. Thus, protein A immunoadsorption fills a critical therapeutic void, particularly in patients with complete tumor remission or minimal residual or recurrent malignant disease.

Antibody Extraction

Another protein A column, still in premarketing trials, has been used to exhaustively adsorb IgG antibodies in patients with coagulation factor inhibitors, HLA antibodies and other specific antibodies. The system consists of two protein A columns (Immunosorba®, purified staphylococcal protein A linked to agarose) and an elution monitor. A cell separator provides plasma to the columns, which are sequentially eluted and regenerated to maximize IgG removal and expand the capacity of the procedure indefinitely. This system was used in 10 highly and persistently sensitized patients awaiting renal transplantation to remove anti-HLA antibodies, resulting in significant reduction of circulating IgG levels, HLA antibody titers and preformed reactive antibody levels. More importantly, of seven patients who received a kidney allograft, only one rejected the allograft.[21]

A second study by Hakim et al[22] in 10 highly sensitized patients awaiting renal transplantation demonstrated reduction of IgG levels by 88 ± 8% with a concomitant reduction in albumin of 11%. Specific anti-HLA antibody titers were reduced by a factor of 12. As in the previous study, no adverse effects were observed clinically or from changes in blood chemistries. The procedure demonstrated a transient and significant reduction of HLA antibodies in patients treated immediately before transplantation. Overall, the tolerance to the procedure has been remarkable in 32 patients treated 161 times with no reactions reported. In one study, C3a levels were studied and no complement activation could be demonstrated. The application of this system should be considered experimental and used only under an appropriately approved protocol.

Cancer

Immunoperfusion technology with protein A was first used in a patient with colon carcinoma in whom a decrease in tumor size, tumoricidal effect and removal of blocking factors were observed.[23] A similar effect was reported by several investigators in patients with breast carcinoma, melanoma and renal adenocarcinoma.[24-26] Toxicity of varying severity was observed in these patients, including fever, chills, pain, bronchospasm, hypotension and death. The initial experience with protein A perfusion was obtained with a variety of protein A preparations linked to various solid matrices in on-line or off-line systems. Under those conditions it is not surprising to find variable tumor responses as well as variable reaction rates. As the technology has evolved, there is now experience with a standardized protein A column, the Prosorba® column.

Recently the results of Phase I and Phase II studies of the experience of the Prosorba® column in a multicenter trial in the United States were reported.[27] A total of 142 patients underwent a total of 1306 treatments.

These 142 patients were eligible for evaluation of toxicity response, and 101 patients were eligible for evaluation of tumor response. The total tumor response rate was 22 patients or 21.8%. Side effects consisted mainly of chills, fever, pain and nausea (28%, 28%, 16% and 10%, respectively). Hypertension, hypotension, headache, joint pain and rash were seen less frequently. This study corroborated initial observations that immunoadsorption with protein A columns can result in tumor response. However, the therapeutic role of protein A column immunoadsorption in oncologic therapy is yet to be defined and its application should be considered experimental.

Mechanism of Action of Immunoaffinity Apheresis

Protein A is a well-known cell wall protein only found in the Cowan I strain of *Staphylococcus aureus*. It is usually released in the surrounding medium, ie, culture medium, and possesses IgG-Fc-receptor functions, which confers to it the affinity to react strongly with human and mammalian IgG subclasses 1, 2 and 4 and more so with antigen-bound IgG, as in circulating immune complexes (CIC). Protein A has been used extensively as an immunologic reagent and studied in great detail with regard to specific isolation of immunoglobulins and immune complexes. In contrast, identification and quantitation of CIC are still fraught with uncertainties. Currently, no single method gives satisfactory information about specificity, size, weight and pathogenic significance of CIC. Such shortcomings preclude complete definition of the pathogenic role of CIC and the relevance of their extraction by immunoadsorption.

Complexed protein A and IgG strongly activate the classical complement pathway and indirectly the alternate pathway in vivo and in vitro.[28] Complement activation is maximum when there is an IgG excess. Protein A also has a mitogenic effect on T and B lymphocytes. Plasma perfused over a column containing protein A becomes mitogenic for lymphocytes, which are thus activated.[29] Soluble preparations of protein A are capable of inducing A and B interferon secretion by mononuclear cells, which is probably the result of some staphylococcal enterotoxin A contamination of the protein A preparations.[30] Singly or combined, these effects could account for the immunologic changes observed during trials of patients with autoimmune or malignant diseases.

It is doubtful that the reported utility of protein A immunoadsorption could be explained by direct removal of platelet-binding IgG and CIC from a patient's plasma, which amounts to as little as 1 mg of CIC and 1 g of IgG. An immunomodulation model based on the removal of IgG-CIC has been proposed to explain the reported therapeutic effect and is based on the immunosuppressive and regulatory effect of CIC.[31] In it, removal of immunosuppressive platelet directed Ig-anti-F(ab')$_2$ CIC [PDIg-anti-F(ab')$_2$ CIC] would trigger a transient depression of anti-F(ab')$_2$ production. Anti-F(ab')$_2$ antibodies may neutralize PDIg and create larger PDIg containing CIC and thus enhance their uptake and clearance by the reticuloendothelial system. Production of large quantities of anti-F(ab')$_2$ may suppress production of auto-idiotypes by a mechanism of idiotypic suppression.[32] Involvement of auto-anti-idiotypes in the regulation of production of specific autoantibodies in patients with autoimmune disease has long been suspected. Removal of platelet-associated IgG and CIC by the protein A column (Prosorba®) has been documented.[31]

In CCATTP/HUS, there is evidence that immunologic factors, particularly CIC, play a role in its pathogenesis. High titers of CIC have been demonstrated in patients with CCATTP/HUS with varying size distribution and properties of platelet aggregating activity, and adenocarcinoma cell and IgG reactivity.[33] While, as pointed out before, the protein column removes IgG and CIC, it is doubtful that this is the sole explanation for its therapeutic effect. Snyder et al (unpublished observations) propose that activation of the complement cascade, stimulation of monocytic and macrophagic cells and production of anti-F(ab')$_2$ antibodies may contribute to the clearance of additional CIC posttreatment. They believe further studies are needed to clarify the precise mechanism by which protein A immunoadsorption induces sustained depletion of CIC.

Activation of the complement cascade with resulting elevated levels of C3a, C4a and C5a has been observed in patients' plasma after treatment with the Prosorba® column.[34] The activated components stimulate activity and growth of immune reactive cells and by binding to CIC stimulate clearance of CIC by the reticuloendothelial system. The effect of protein A immunoadsorption is initially characterized by an increase of cells of the granulocyte and macrophage lineage, followed by lymphocyte increase with increased blastogenic response to mitogens and elevation of the T helper/suppressor cell ratio and increased natural killer cell activity. There is also a striking increase in antibody against disease associated antigens with antigen/antibody ratio changing from antigen excess to antibody excess posttreatment. This results in modulation of immune responses against disease-related antigens, which has been demonstrated in animal and in human experiments.[34]

The Prosorba® column removes CIC containing specific antibody and Le^X glycolipid antigens from plasma of patients with breast adenocarcinoma.[35] Following protein A treatment, patients with breast carcinoma produced increasing amounts of anti-Le^X antibodies. This, in turn, led to an increased recruitment of free Le^X antigen into CIC, resulting in an increased uptake and removal of the tumor-associated Le^X glycolipids from the circulating pool. Interestingly enough, the patients who demonstrated the greatest increases in specific antibody production were those who also experienced objective antitumor responses. This suggested that a mechanism of antitumor action may be the induction of tumor-specific antibody formation in patients with breast adenocarcinoma. Thus, it would appear that protein A immunoadsorption acts as a biologic response modifier.

However, further research is needed to achieve a complete understanding of the precise mechanism of action of protein A immunoadsorption in autoimmune disease and cancer.

Complement activation by the Prosorba® column possibly explains its therapeutic effect as well as some of its toxicity. Experimental models of protein columns are charting a new course by abandoning the use of the staphylococcal protein A and adopting a recombinant material as well as a different carrier. A new experimental system that is also capable of activating complement uses an attachment to absorb the activated compounds, which are thus prevented from reaching the patient's circulation. It would be of great interest to determine whether or not the new column has the same therapeutic effect or no effect to either confirm or deny the therapeutic value of the activated complement compounds. The toxicity of the new column is likely to better define the participation of the complement activated components in the pathogenesis of the reactions associated with protein A immunoadsorption.

Summary

In all likelihood, we will continue to witness the evolution of what promises to be an exciting and dynamic endeavor in the therapeutic selective extraction of plasma constituents. A wider application of existing technology is expected, possibly with a greater variety of sorbents and carriers. The production of new monoclonal antibodies and recombinant synthesis of biomaterials create new opportunities to selectively extract undesirable elements to achieve a therapeutic goal. Technology is not the limiting factor but rather the uncertainty about the pathogenic properties of the plasma constituent to be removed. In this regard, the new techniques have contributed already and will do so in the future to expand our understanding of disease pathogenesis.

References

1. Pineda AA. Selective plasma component removal. Mount Kisco, NY: Futura, 1984.
2. Pineda AA. Future directions of apheresis. In: Valbonesi M, Pineda AA, Biggs JC, eds. Therapeutic hemapheresis. Milano: Wichtig Editore, 1986:187-94.
3. Saal SD, Parker TS, Gordon BR, et al. Removal of low-density lipoproteins in patients by extracorporeal immunoadsorption. Am J Med 1986;80:583-9.
4. Buffaloe GW, Erickson RR, Dau PC. Evaluation of a parallel plate membrane plasma exchange system. J Clin Apheresis 1983;1:86-94.

5. Agishi T, Amemiya H, Ota K, Sugino N. Usefulness of double filtration plasmapheresis in comparison with standard centrifugation plasmapheresis. In: Nose Y, Malchesky PS, Smith JW, eds. Plasmapheresis. Cleveland: ISAO Press, 1983:127-32.

6. Krakauer RS, Asanuma Y, Zawicki J, et al. Circulating immune complexes in rheumatoid arthritis: Selective removal by cryogelation with membrane filtration. Arch Intern Med 1982;142:395-7.

7. Young JB, Ayus JC, Miller LK, et al. Cardiopulmonary toxicity in patients with breast carcinoma during plasma perfusion over immobilized protein A. Am J Med 1983;75:278-88.

8. Terman DS, Bertram JH. Antitumor effects of immobilized protein A and staphylococcal products: Linkage between toxicity and efficacy, identification of potential tumoricidal reagents. Eur J Cancer Clin Oncol 1985;21:1115-22.

9. Smith EM, Johnson HM, Blaylock JE. Staphylococcal protein A induces the production of interferon-α in human lymphocytes and interferon-α in mouse spleen cells. J Immunol 1983;130:773-6.

10. Kinet JP, Hunt J, Foidart JB, et al. Ex vivo perfusion of plasma over protein A columns in human mammary adenocarcinoma. Evidence for a protein A leaking by radioimmunoassay. Eur J Clin Invest 1986;16:43-9.

11. Korec S, Smith FP, Schein PS, Phillips TM. Clinical experiences with extracorporeal immunoperfusions of plasma from cancer patients. J Biol Response Mod 1984;3:330-5.

12. Terman DS. Preparation of protein A immobilized on collodion-coated charcoal and plasma perfusion system for treatment of cancer. Method Enzymol 1988;137:496-515.

13. Jones FR, Balint JR Jr, Snyder HW Jr. The Prosorba column clinical trial group: selective extracorporeal removal of immunoglobulin-G and circulating immune complexes. Plasma Ther Transfus Technol 1986;7:333-49.

14. Garey DC, Perry E, Jackson B. Fatal pulmonary reaction with staph protein A immune adsorption for pure red cell aplasia. (abstract). Transfusion 1988;28:245.

15. Mittelman A, Bertram JH, Henry DH, et al. Treatment of patients with HIV thrombocytopenia and hemolytic uremic syndrome (HUS) with protein A column (Prosorba® column) immunoadsorption. Semin Hematol 1989;26:15-18.

16. Guthrie TH Jr. Immune thrombocytopenia purpura: A pilot study of staphylococcal protein A immunomodulation in refractory patients. Semin Hematol 1989;26:3-9.

17. Muroi K, Sasaki R, Miura Y. The effect of immunoadsorption therapy by a protein A column on patients with thrombocytopenia. Semin Hematol 1989;26:10-14.

18. Korec S, Schein PS, Smith PF, et al. Treatment of cancer-associated hemolytic uremic syndrome with staphylococcal protein A immunoperfusion. J Clin Oncol 1986;4:210-5.
19. Sheldon R, Slougher D. A syndrome of microangiopathic hemolytic anemia, renal impairment, and pulmonary edema in chemotherapy-treated patients with adenocarcinoma. Cancer 1986;58:1428-36.
20. Murgo AS. Thrombotic microangiopathy in the cancer patient including those induced by chemotherapeutic agents. Semin Hematol 1987;24:161-77.
21. Palmer A, Taube D, Welsh K, et al. Removal of anti-HLA antibodies by extracorporeal immunoadsorption to enable renal transplantation. Lancet 1989;1:10-2.
22. Hakim RM, Milford E, Himmelfarb J, et al. Extracorporeal removal of anti-HLA antibodies in transplant candidates. Am J Kidney Dis 1990;16:423-31.
23. Bansal SC, Bansal BR, Thomas HL. Ex-vivo removal of serum IgG in a patient with colon carcinoma. Cancer 1978;42:1-18.
24. Terman DS, Young JB, Shearer WT. Preliminary observations of the effects on breast adenocarcinoma of plasma perfused over immobilized protein A. N Engl J Med 1981;305:1195-200.
25. Bensinger WI, Kinet JP, Hennen G, et al. Plasma perfused over immobilized protein A for breast cancer. N Engl J Med 1982;306:935-6.
26. Hakansson L, Jonsson S, Sodeberg M, et al. Tumor regression after extracorporeal affinity chromatography of blood plasma across agarose beads containing staphylococcal protein A. Eur J Cancer Clin Oncol 1984;20:1377-88.
27. Messerschmidt GL, Henry DH, Snyder HW, et al. Protein A immunotherapy in the treatment of cancer: An update. Semin Hematol 1989;26:19-24.
28. Langone JJ, Boyle MDP, Borsos T. Studies on the interaction between protein A and immunoglobulin G. II. Composition and activity of complexes formed between protein A and IgG. J Immunol 1978; 121:333.
29. Bertram JH, Hengst JCD, Mitchell MS. Staphylococcal protein A immunoadsorptive column induces mitogenicity in perfused plasma. J Biol Response Mod 1984;3:235.
30. Ratliff TL, McCool RE, Catalona WJ. Interferon induction and augmentation of natural-killer activity by staphylococcus protein A. Cell Immunol 1981;57:1.
31. Snyder HW Jr, Bertram JH, Channel M, et al. Reduction in platelet-binding immunoglobulins and improvement in platelet counts in patients with HIV-associated idiopathic thrombocytopenic purpura (ITP) following extracorporeal immunoadsorption of plasma over staphylococcal protein A-silica. Artif Organs 1988;13:71-7.

32. Burdette S, Schwartz RS. Idiotypes and idiotypic networks. N Engl J Med 1987;317:219.

33. Zimmerman SE, Smith FP, Phillips TM, et al. Gastric carcinoma and thrombotic thrombocytopenic purpura: Association with plasma immune complex concentrations. Br Med J 1982;284:1432-4.

34. Snyder HW Jr, Belint JP Jr, Jones FR. Modulation of immunity in patients with autoimmune disease and cancer treated by extracorporeal immunoadsorption with Prosorba® columns. Semin Hematol 1989;26:31-41.

35. Singhal AK, Singhal MC, Nudelman E, et al. Presence of fucolipid antigens with mono and dimeric X determinant (Le^x) in the circulating immune complexes of patients with adenocarcinoma. Cancer Res 1989:47;5566-71.

In: Sacher RA, Brubaker DB, Kasprisin DO and McCarthy LJ, eds.
Cellular and Humoral Immunotherapy and Apheresis
Arlington, VA: American Association of Blood Banks, 1991

4

Redirecting Nature's Toxins To Treat Lymphoma

Ellen S. Vitetta, PhD

A LONG SOUGHT-AFTER GOAL in the treatment of disseminated malignant disease is selective elimination of tumor cells
without damage to normal tissues. Currently, treatments generally
utilize agents that affect dividing cells, both normal and malignant, and
hence produce major side effects.

In the past two decades, predominantly through the development of
monoclonal antibody technology,[1] selective targeting of tumor cells has
been explored as a modality for treating those cancers in which specific
markers on tumor cells can be identified. Thousands of monoclonal antibodies that recognize markers on a variety of tumor cells have been
developed worldwide. When these monoclonal antibodies are administered to animals or humans, they bind to the tumor cells. However,
targeting of antibodies alone is usually insufficient to achieve the extent
of tumor cell destruction required. Because of this, investigators have
attached drugs, toxins, isotopes and other agents to these antibodies to
selectively deliver cytotoxic agents to the tumor cells. While the results
of such approaches have been encouraging, "tagged" antibodies often
perform less efficiently in vivo than would have been predicted from
results in vitro. There has been a need, therefore, to understand the in
vivo behavior of these biological missiles and to optimize strategies for
their use. Efforts have focused on the targeting of toxins to cancer cells
and, in particular, B-cell lymphoma cells. The antibody-toxin molecules
(immunotoxins) have undergone more than a decade of study since their
initial description in 1979-80.[2] Thus, first-generation immunotoxins were

Ellen S. Vitetta, PhD, Professor of Microbiology, Department of Microbiology and
Director, Cancer Immunobiology Center, University of Texas Southwestern Medical
Center, Dallas, Texas
(This work is supported by NIH grants CA28149, CA41081, AI21229 and a grant from
the Welch Foundation.)

refined into second-generation versions, which have greatly improved antitumor effects. Second-generation immunotoxins are currently being tested in humans. While it is too early to predict their long-range impact on cancer therapy, early results are encouraging. This chapter will describe the development of immunotoxins, the problems in improving them and their current clinical performance.

Immunotoxins

Immunotoxins usually consist of tumor-cell-reactive monoclonal antibodies covalently coupled to natural or genetically engineered toxins or their toxic subunits.[3] Each component of the immunotoxin—antibody, toxin and the chemical linker used to bind the antibody to the toxin—plays a critical role in its specificity, toxicity and in vivo behavior.

Monoclonal Antibodies

Monoclonal antibodies of rodent or human origin can be generated by fusing precursors of antibody-forming B lymphocytes from immunized humans or rodents to immortalized myeloma cells.[1] One parent cell (the B cell) confers antibody specificity and the other (the myeloma cell) confers immortality on the "hybridoma." Hy-bridomas are grown in media that do not allow the survival of the parent cells; the media from the hybridomas are then screened to select clones that secrete antibodies of the desired specificity, affinity and immunoglobulin isotype. These clones can be maintained in culture or in animals where they divide and secrete large quantities of the desired monoclonal antibody. Monoclonal antibodies can then be purified and used in their native form or fragmented into smaller portions containing only their antigen-binding segments. In the past several years, hybridoma technology has evolved to utilize the techniques of modern molecular biology to introduce human sequences into murine antibody and to create antibodies of higher affinity.[4] In addition, RNA or DNA encoding antibody-combining regions have been extracted from B cells and cDNA or gDNA libraries have been expressed in a variety of cells, including bacteria.[5] The transfected cells are then screened and selected for production of antibodies of the desired specificity.

Specificity of Monoclonal Antibodies

In general, immunotoxins prepared from antibodies directed against tumor-associated antigens kill not only the tumor cells, but also nonneoplastic cells of the same lineage. In certain instances, this is acceptable. For example, the killing of normal lymphocytes can be tolerated because lymphocytes are constantly being regenerated from marrow progenitor cells. In other instances, destruction of nonneoplastic cells of the same lineage is unacceptable, eg, cells of the nervous system, which regenerate slowly, if at all. It should be emphasized that a minor cross-reaction with a life-sustaining normal tissue, which might be overlooked when screening an unconjugated antibody, can lead to major toxicity when that monoclonal antibody is attached to a toxin.

Antibody Fragments

It is currently unclear which particular forms of cancer (or any other diseases) will benefit from using the intact antibody molecule as opposed to an antibody fragment as the carrier of a toxin. On the one hand, Fab' and F(ab')$_2$ fragments of antibody are less immunogenic and, lacking the Fc portion, cannot bind to cells via their Fc receptors. Furthermore, they are smaller than intact antibody and their decreased size may be advantageous for penetration into solid tumor masses. On the other hand, antibody fragments are more rapidly cleared from the blood and tissues than are intact antibodies and so have less time to reach their target cells.[6,7] Also, Fab'/Fab fragments bind to their target cells less avidly than their bivalent counterparts and are usually less potent in vitro.[8,9]

Immunogenicity

Another important consideration in the use of antibodies as targeting vehicles is their immunogenicity. Antibody responses are usually generated to both the antibody and toxin components, thus rendering them ineffective after one or two courses of therapy.[10] This precludes the repeated use of immunotoxins in clinical trials. Besides the obvious strategy of treating patients who are already immunosuppressed because of their disease (eg, lymphoma), various immunosuppressive regimens have been employed during therapy to prevent the generation of antibody responses.[10] It is not known, however, whether immunosuppression will be beneficial to the final outcome of therapy; it is possible that after the majority of tumor cells have been eliminated by immunotoxins, an immune response may be necessary to keep remaining viable tumor cells in check. A recent strategy to avoid the use of immunosuppressive agents, yet prevent an immune response to the antibody component of the immunotoxin, has been to "humanize" the antibody by genetic engineering.[4,11,12] Humanizing antibodies represents a sound strategy to avoid an immune response to the antibody but is unlikely to affect the immune response to the toxin.

The Toxin Portion of an Immunotoxin

Thus far, the toxins that have been used to form immunotoxins are derived from bacteria or plants and are inhibitors of protein synthesis.[13] These toxins consist of subunits or domains that mediate cell binding, membrane translocation and enzymatic (toxic) activity. Natural toxins are among the most powerful cell poisons and it is estimated that fewer than 10 molecules will kill a cell if it enters the cytosol (although many times that number must bind to the cell surface because the entry process is inefficient).[14-16] This extraordinary potency initially led to the concern that such poisons were too powerful to control. However, as discussed below, the nonspecific toxicity of the toxins can be markedly reduced by removing or modifying their cell-binding domain or subunit. The remaining portion of the toxin (lacking a cell-binding domain) is then coupled to an antibody that targets the toxic portion to the cancer cell. By selecting an antibody lacking unwanted cross-reactivity, immunotoxins are safer and have far fewer nonspecific cytotoxic effects than conventional anticancer drugs. Another attraction of toxins is that because they are inhibitors of protein synthesis, they can kill resting cells as efficiently as dividing cells. Hence, tumor cells that are not in cycle at the time of treatment do not escape the cytotoxic effect of an immunotoxin.

Ricin and Its A Chain

The most frequently used plant toxin is ricin. Ricin is synthesized in the endosperm of the caster bean as a single polypeptide chain and is then processed posttranslationally to yield the mature toxin composed of two disulfide-bonded subunits, A and B.[13] The B chain is a galactose-specific lectin that binds to glycoproteins and glycolipids present on the surface of all cell types in higher animals. After binding, the toxin enters the cell by endocytosis and the A chain (which contains translocation and enzymatic domains) is translocated across the membrane of an intracellular vesicle into the cytosol by a poorly understood process. The A chain is released from the B chain by reduction and kills the cell by catalytically removing an adenine residue from the ribosomal 60S subunit, which is necessary for the binding of elongation factor 2 (EF2).[14,15]

Preparation of Immunotoxins

Disulfide Linkage

For in vivo therapy, the antibody and ricin toxin A chain must be coupled in such a way as to remain stable while passing through the bloodstream and the tissues, yet be labile within the target cell so that the toxic portion can be released into the cytosol. There have been extensive reviews on the preparation and purification of immunotoxins using different types of linkers.[17]

Linkers used to couple intact IgG to ricin A chain introduce a disulfide bond between the ligand and A chain. Bonds that cannot be reduced (eg, thioether bonds) render these immunotoxins either much less toxic or nontoxic,[9] suggesting that the A chain is released from the ligand by intracellular reduction. The linker used to couple the A chain to the ligand is usually a heterobifunctional cross-linker that introduces an activated thiol group into the antibody. The thiolated antibody is then mixed with the reduced A chain and disulfide change occurs to create an antibody-A chain conjugate. In the case of Fab' and some Fab fragments of antibodies there is a free cysteine residue near the hinge region, which can be used to form a disulfide bridge with the free cysteine residue of the A chain.[6] The coupling is generally accomplished by activating the thiol group in the Fab'/Fab fragment with Ellman's reagent[18] (to provide a good leaving group) and mixing the derivatized Fab'/Fab with the reduced A chain. The Fab'/Fab-A then forms by a thiol-disulfide exchange reaction. Since the thiol group of the Fab'/Fab fragment is distant from its antigen-combining site and since there is usually only one free thiol group on the fragments derived from most subclasses of monoclonal antibodies, the attachment of one A chain per Fab'/Fab fragment at a site distant from the combining site is ensured. Such constructs retain full antigen-binding activity unlike IgG-As and Fab-As that are constructed using cross-linkers that can introduce the A chain in or near the combining site of an antibody in a proportion of the molecules.[8]

First-Generation Cross-Linkers

The "first-generation" heterobifunctional cross-linkers [ie, 3-(2-pyridyl-dithio) propionic acid N-hydroxysuccinimide ester] (SPDP) generated disulfide bonds that were relatively unstable in vivo and released A chain and antibody with a T½ of 6-8 hours.[6,19,20] The breakdown is probably due to reduction by glutathione, albumin and other thiol-containing mole-cules in the blood and tissues. This problem has been solved by the synthesis of new cross-linkers (eg, SMPT[20,21]), which introduce hindered disulfide bonds having phenyl and/or methyl groups adjacent to the disulfide bond. Immunotoxins prepared with these hindered cross-linkers are much more stable (T½ approximately 2 days) and have improved antitumor activities.[21]

Cytotoxic Properties of Immunotoxins

Ricin A chain-containing immunotoxins show virtually complete specificity in their cytotoxic effect upon target cells in vitro because their only means of binding to cells is by their antibody portion. Fc binding, if it occurs, appears not to route the immunotoxin to an intracellular compartment favorable for A chain release and cell killing. The major disadvantage of these immunotoxins is their variable cytotoxic potencies; some have little or none, whereas others are highly potent.[22-24]

It is now generally accepted that the binding avidity of the antibody plays a major role in determining whether or not it will become an effective immunotoxin.[8,23,25,26] Those antibodies with low binding affinities generally make poor immunotoxins, whereas those with high affinities are usually good. This is probably the main reason why Fab'-As, having only one antigen-combining site, tend to be 3-100 times less effective than their intact antibody counterparts, which have high avidities because of their bivalency. In addition, the cell surface molecule that the antibody recognizes plays a key role in determining the efficacy of the immunotoxin.[24,27,28] In general, cell surface molecules that continuously recycle into endosomal compartments (eg, growth factor receptors) or that can be induced to do so by binding to an antibody or other ligand, make effective targets for immunotoxins. Cell surface molecules that are not readily internalized or that are internalized into intracellular compartments unfavorable for A chain translocation (eg, the lysosomes) make poor immunotoxins no matter how high the avidity of the antibody. More recently, it has been reported that the target antigen, which is often a large cell surface glycoprotein, can have numerous epitopes and that antibodies against different epitopes can differ in their effectiveness as immunotoxins.[24,28] The most likely explanation for this is that antibodies may have to recognize epitopes close to the plasma membrane for the A chain to insert into the membrane and be translocated across the membrane and into the cytosol after endocytosis.[27,28]

Since only a minority of monoclonal antibodies make potent immunotoxins, an assay has been developed to screen monoclonal antibodies to predict which ones will make effective immunotoxins.[29] This assay involves binding the antibody (in the form of a tissue culture supernatant or ascites) to target cells and then treating the coated cells with a secondary Fab' or Fab fragment of an anti-mouse, anti-rat or anti-human Ig linked to an A chain. The degree of killing achieved predicts quite accurately the potency of that antibody as an A chain immunotoxin. This assay represents an important development since previously, each antibody had to undergo time-consuming purification, linkage to the A chain and evaluation by cytotoxicity assays on target cells.

Tissue Distribution and Toxicology of Immunotoxins in Rodents

Ricin A chain is glycosylated and contains mannose- and fucose-terminating oligosaccharides.[30] These sugars are recognized by avid receptors on both the parenchymal and nonparenchymal cells in the liver.[31,32] Hence, immunotoxins prepared from native A chain are cleared rapidly from the blood. This may have been at least partially responsible for the failure of first-generation immunotoxins to reach target cells in vivo and elicit their antitumor effects.

The problem of liver recognition of ricin or its A chain was solved by destroying ["deglycosylating" (dgA)] the mannose and fucose residues in the holotoxin by a simple procedure involving periodate oxidation and cyanoborohydride reduction at low pH.[33] This procedure does not affect the enzymatic activity of the A chain or its ability to function as part of an immunotoxin. Immunotoxins prepared with dgA, intact antibodies and stable linkers are long-lived in vivo[20,21]: in mice lacking target cells for which they are specific, the immunotoxin is cleared only twice as rapidly as native IgG.

At doses of dgA containing immunotoxins approaching the LD_{50}, tissue damage in mice and primates is observed in the crypts of Leiberkuhn, the small intestine, the proximal tubules of the kidney and in skeletal muscle.[34,35] None of these effects appears sufficiently severe to cause death. The cause of death at high doses is unknown. Fab'-immunotoxins induce similar toxic side effects except that in some experiments myositis is more marked, possibly because they permeate extravascular tissues more readily because of their smaller size. On the other hand, the LD_{50} of Fab'-immunotoxins is 3-5 times greater on a total protein basis (ie, less toxic) than that of IgG-immunotoxins, probably because the former are more rapidly cleared.[6]

The Performance of Immunotoxins in Animals

It has been established in animals that marked antitumor effects, prolonged remissions and even cures can be achieved with doses of immunotoxins that are well-tolerated.[36-42] In general, tumors that are accessible to the circulation (ie, lymphoma and leukemia) appear to be most responsive[42] but impressive regressions of large, solid tumors have also been reported. In addition, the effectiveness of this therapy in conjunction with conventional therapy has been well-documented in animals. For example, access of immunotoxins to solid tumors and antitumor activity can be improved by co-administration of β-adrenergic blockers, which may act by selectively constricting normal vasculature and increasing the tumor-to-normal tissue perfusion ratio.[43] Chemotherapy and immunotoxin therapy have a synergistic effect.[44]

"Cocktails" of immunotoxins are superior to a single immunotoxin because antigen-deficient tumor cell mutants can escape killing and grow as the dominant clone if only a single immunotoxin has been used.[21,41] Mutant tumor cells that express the target antigen, but fail to transport the toxic component of the immunotoxin to the cytosol can also emerge, albeit less frequently than the antigen-deficient mutants. It will probably be necessary to administer immunotoxins in combination with conventional chemotherapeutic drugs or radiotherapy. Because the modes of action of the different therapies do not overlap, the resistant mutants that escape one type of therapy may succumb to another.

Cytoreductive therapy and immunotoxin therapy together may reduce a tumor burden to a level where the immune system of the host can suppress the growth of the remaining tumor cells.[37,45] This is analogous to the human situation where remissions may last for several years before the dormant tumor cells begin to divide at a rapid rate and relapse occurs. These findings emphasize that it may not be necessary to kill every tumor cell in order to induce a prolonged remission *if* the immune system is functional.

The administration of immunotoxins to animals with an intact immune system leads to an antibody response against both components of the immunotoxin, precluding repeated treatments. Immunosuppressive regimens can delay anti-immunotoxin responses but may also compromise the host's ability to suppress the growth of residual tumor. Until specific tolerance to an immunotoxin can be achieved it will be necessary to administer them in a short course prior to the development of a primary antibody response.

Animal studies have facilitated the evaluation and refinement of different types of immunotoxin constructs. First-generation immunotoxins containing native A chain and unstable linkers were altered to generate second-generation versions. These contain dgA and stable linkers and they have dramatically superior antitumor activity compared to their predecessors. Fab'-immunotoxins have been compared with IgG-immunotoxins and, depending on the test system, have weaker or equivalent antitumor activity but lower immunogenicity.

Clinical Trials in Humans

First-Generation Immunotoxins

The results of clinical trials with first-generation immunotoxins were disappointing.[46-49] This can be attributed to several factors beyond the obvious problem of attempting to treat large, refractory tumors in typical

Phase I dose escalation protocols. First-generation immunotoxins containing native A chain had, as described previously, some predictable side effects such as binding to liver cells, which reduced their ability to reach tumor sites effectively. Initially, it was not appreciated that the cytotoxic potency of many of the immunotoxins was not optimal. Second, some of the tumors treated (ie, melanoma and breast carcinoma) were probably not ideal tumors to treat since solid tumors are not readily accessible to the systemic circulation. In the case of accessible tumors such as chronic lymphocytic leukemia, the majority of the circulating tumor cells failed to internalize the immunotoxin effectively.[49] In these trials it was not determined whether the target antigen was on the progenitor cells. It has also become apparent that antibody responses that were seen in animals are a major problem in humans whose disease or former therapy is not immunosuppressive.[10] Maneuvers to avoid an anti-immunotoxin response are being tested and must succeed before repeated courses of therapy can be given. Until this is accomplished, immunotoxins will have to be administered as a single course of therapy; this will reduce their utility in cancer therapy, except in treating minimal disease.

Despite these problems, tumor regressions were seen in some patients for whom all other therapies had failed.[47,48] These responses were generally transient and did not meet World Health Organization criteria. Nevertheless, as noted above, it must be appreciated that these responses were achieved in situations where patients carried enormous tumor burdens, and often had underlying conditions from prior therapy that predisposed them to toxicity. None of these trials has reached Phase III. Instead, second-generation constructs are currently being tested in Phase I/II trials with the intention of using them to treat minimal residual disease and metastases, either alone or in combination with conventional therapy.

The major dose-limiting side effect of immunotoxins observed in the clinical trials was vascular leak syndrome (VLS).[10] The manifestations of this syndrome are extravasation of albumin and other proteins into the extravascular space, retention of water in the peripheral tissues and weight gains, which, in some cases, can lead to pulmonary edema and other life-threatening situations. In addition, side effects such as malaise, low-grade fever, myalgias and tachycardia were common; as with VLS, these had not been predicted from studies in mice or monkeys. The causes of these side effects have not been determined, although they may involve release of cytokines and damage to vascular endothelial cells. Since VLS is a major side effect of interleukin-2 and γ-interferon therapy as well,[50,51] it is likely that cytokines are involved in immunotoxin-mediated VLS. It is now necessary to go back to animal studies in order to determine the cause and prevention of VLS and related side effects.

It became apparent from treating patients with tumors that immunotoxins might be more advantageous, at least as first-generation reagents, in treating diseases where cells are more accessible to the bloodstream, where mutants are less frequent and where every cell does not have to be killed to achieve a beneficial effect. Thus, immunotoxins that kill normal T cells have shown considerable efficacy in the treatment of steroid-resis tant graft-vs-host disease [52,53] (caused by allogeneic bone marrow transplantation) and, more recently, in autoimmune disorders.[54] Since results of these applications are more encouraging, immunotoxins are currently being considered for the therapy of viral diseases, inflammatory diseases, allergies, parasitic infections and other dysfunctions where cells of the immune system can be targeted. Therefore, despite their suboptimal performance as antitumor drugs, immunotoxins have now found a possible application in the treatment of a variety of other diseases where they may prove highly efficacious.

Second-Generation Immunotoxins

Results of Phase I clinical trials with second-generation Fab'- and IgG-immunotoxins containing stable linkers and deglycosylated A chain are encouraging.[55] While VLS remains the major side effect, liver damage has not occurred. The antitumor effect of these immunotoxins in lymphoma has been encouraging, with a 40-50% response rate. When these immunotoxins are used at safe doses in Phase II trials, it is expected that the antitumor response rate should be higher.

The challenge of eradicating cancer cells is a formidable one and cancer represents a heterogeneous collection of disease states. It is not unexpected, therefore, that the transfer of technology from the laboratory to the clinic has also been challenging. We are in the early stages of clinical trials but the results are encouraging. Strategies necessary to solve the current problems are emerging and will be incorporated into future clinical trials.

Acknowledgments

I thank Ms. D. Thomas for secretarial assistance and Dr. J. Uhr for helpful comments concerning the writing of this review.

References

1. Köhler G, Milstein C. Continuous cultures of fused cells secreting antibody of predefined specificity. Nature 1975;256:495-7.
2. Möller G, ed. Antibody carriers of drugs and toxins in tumor therapy. Immunol Rev 1982;62:1-216.
3. Vitetta ES, Fulton RJ, May RD, et al. Redesigning nature's poisons to create anti-tumor reagents. Science 1987;238:1098-104.
4. Winter G, Milstein C. Man-made antibodies. Nature 1991;349:293-9.

5. Ward ES, Güssow D, Griffith AD, et al. Binding activities of repertoire of single immunoglobulin variable domains secreted from *Escherichia coli*. Nature 1989;341:544-6.

6. Fulton RJ, Tucker TF, Vitetta ES, et al. Pharmacokinetics of tumor-reactive immunotoxins in tumor-bearing mice: Effect of antibody valency and deglycosylation of the ricin A chain on clearance and tumor localization. Cancer Res 1988;48:2618-25.

7. Holton OD III, Black CDV, Parker RJ, et al. Biodistribution of monoclonal IgG_1, $F(ab')_2$ and Fab' in mice after intravenous injection. Comparison between anti-B cell (anti-LyB8.2) and irrelevant (MOPC21) antibodies. J Immunol 1987;39:3041-9.

8. Ghetie M-A, May RD, Till M, et al. Evaluation of ricin A chain-containing immunotoxins directed against CD19 and CD22 antigens on normal and malignant human B-cells as potential reagents for in vivo therapy. Cancer Res 1988;48:2610-17.

9. Masuho Y, Kishida K, Saito M, et al. Importance of the antigen-binding valency and the nature of cross-linking bond in ricin A chain conjugates with antibody. J Biochem 1982;91:1583-91.

10. Byers VS, Baldwin RW. Therapeutic strategies with monoclonal antibodies and immunoconjugates. Immunol 1988;65:329-35.

11. Morrison SL, Johnson MJ, Herzenberg LA, et al. Chimeric human antibody molecules: Mouse antigen-binding domains with human constant region domains. Proc Natl Acad Sci (USA) 1984;81:6851-5.

12. Shaw DR, Khazaeli MB, Lobuglio AF. Biological activity of mouse/human chimeric antibodies of the four human IgG subclasses with specificity for a tumor-associated antigen. Proc Am Assoc Cancer Res 1988;29:421.

13. Olsnes S, Pihl A. Toxic lectins and related proteins. In: Cohen P, van Heyningen S, eds. Molecular action of toxins and viruses. New York: Elsevier, 1982:51-105.

14. Eiklid K, Olsnes S, Pihl A. Entry of lethal doses of abrin, ricin and modeccin into the cytosol of HeLa cells. Exp Cell Res 1980;126:321-6.

15. Endo Y, Mitsui K, Motizuki M, et al. The mechanism of action of ricin and related toxic lectins on eukaryotic ribosomes. The site and the characteristics of the modification in 28 S ribosomal RNA caused by the toxins. J Biol Chem 1987;262:5908-12.

16. Olsnes S, Sandvig K. Entry of polypeptide toxins into animal cells. In: Pastan I, Willingham MC, eds. Endocytosis. New York: Plenum Press, 1988:195-234.

17. Wawrzynczak EJ, Thorpe PE. Methods for preparing immunotoxins: Effects of the linkage on activity and stability. In: Vogel CW, ed. Immunoconjugates: Antibody conjugates in radioimaging and therapy of cancer. New York: Oxford University Press, 1987:28-55.

18. Ellman GL. Tissue sulfhydryl groups. Arch Biochem Biophys 1959; 82:70-7.

19. Blakey DC, Watson GJ, Knowles PP, et al. Effect of chemical deglycosylation of ricin A chain on the in vivo fate and cytotoxic activity of an immunotoxin composed of ricin A chain and anti-Thy 1.1 antibody. Cancer Res 1987;47:947-52.
20. Thorpe PE, Wallace PM, Knowles PP, et al. New coupling agents for the synthesis of immunotoxins containing a hindered disulfide bond with improved stability in vivo. Cancer Res 1987;47:5924-31.
21. Thorpe PE, Wallace PM, Knowles PP, et al. Improved anti-tumor effects of immunotoxins prepared with deglycosylated ricin A chain and hindered disulfide linkages. Cancer Res 1988;48:6396-403.
22. Bjorn MJ, Ring D, Frankel A. Evaluation of monoclonal antibodies for the development of breast cancer immunotoxins. Cancer Res 1985;45:1214-21.
23. Shen G-L, Li J-L, Ghetie M-A, et al. Evaluation of four CD22 antibodies as ricin A chain-containing immunotoxins for the in vivo therapy of human B-cell leukemias and lymphomas. Int J Cancer 1988; 42:792-7.
24. Press OW, Martin P, Thorpe PE, et al. Ricin A-chain containing immunotoxins directed against different epitopes on the CD2 molecule differ in their ability to kill normal and malignant T cells. J Immunol 1988;141:4410-17.
25. Ramakrishnan S, Houston LL. Comparison of the selective cytotoxic effects of immunotoxins containing ricin A chain or pokeweed antiviral protein and anti-Thy 1.1 monoclonal antibodies. Cancer Res 1984;44:201-8.
26. Engert A, Burrows F, Jung WE, et al. Evaluation of ricin A chain-containing immunotoxins directed against CD30 as potential reagents for the treatment of Hodgkin's disease. Cancer Res 1990;50:84-8.
27. Press OW, Vitetta ES, Farr AG, et al. Evaluation of ricin A-chain immunotoxins directed against human T cells. Cell Immunol 1986; 102:10-20.
28. May RD, Finkelman F, Uhr JW, et al. Evaluation of ricin A chain-containing immunotoxins directed against different epitopes on the delta chain of sIgD on murine B cells. J Immunol 1990;144:3637-42.
29. Till M, May RD, Uhr JW, et al. An assay that predicts the ability of monoclonal antibodies to form potent ricin A chain-containing immunotoxins. Cancer Res 1988;48:1119-23.
30. Kimura Y, Hase S, Kobayashi Y, et al. Structures of sugar chains of ricin D. J Biochem (Tokyo) 1988;103:944-9.
31. Blakey DC, Skilleter DN, Price RJ, et al. Uptake of native and deglycosylated ricin A-chain immunotoxins by mouse liver parenchymal and non-parenchymal cells in vitro and in vivo. Biochim Biophys Acta 1988;968:172-8.
32. Skilleter DN, Paine AJ, Stirpe F. A comparison of the accumulation of ricin by hepatic parenchymal and non-parenchymal cells and its

inhibition of protein synthesis. Biochim Biophys Acta 1981;677:495-500.

33. Thorpe PE, Detre SI, Foxwell BMJ, et al. Modification of the carbohydrate in ricin with metaperiodate-cyanoborohydride mixtures. Effects on toxicity and in vivo distribution. Eur J Biochem 1985; 147:197-206.

34. Jansen FK, Blythman HE, Carriere D, et al. Immunotoxins: Hybrid molecules combining high specificity and potent cytotoxicity. Immunol Rev 1982;62:1-85.

35. Soler-Rodriguez AM, Uhr JW, Richardson J, et al. The toxicity of chemically deglycosylated ricin A-chain in mice. Toxicon (In Press).

36. Thorpe PE, Brown AN, Bremner JA Jr, et al. An immunotoxin composed of monoclonal anti-Thy 1.1 antibody and a ribosome-inactivating protein from *Saponaria officinalis*: Potent antitumor effects in vitro and in vivo. J Natl Cancer Inst 1985;75:151-9.

37. Krolick KA, Uhr JW, Slavin S, et al. In vivo therapy of a murine B cell tumor (BCL₁) using antibody-ricin A chain immunotoxins. J Exp Med 1982;155:1797-809.

38. Jansen FK, Blythman HE, Carriere D, et al. High specific cytotoxicity of antibody-toxin hybrid molecules (immunotoxins) for target cells. Immunol Lett 1980;2:97-102.

39. Hara H, Luo Y, Haruta Y, et al. Efficient transplantation of human non-T-leukemia cells into nude mice and induction of complete regression of the transplanted distinct tumors by ricin A-chain conjugates of monoclonal antibodies SN5 and SN6. Cancer Res 1988;48: 4673-80.

40. Ramakrishnan S, Bjorn MJ, Houston LL. Recombinant ricin A chain conjugated to monoclonal antibodies: Improved tumor cell inhibition in the presence of lysosomotropic compounds. Cancer Res 1989; 49:613-17.

41. Thorpe PE, Blakey DC, Brown AN, et al. Comparison of two anti-Thy 1.1-abrin A-chain immunotoxins prepared with different cross-linking agents: Antitumor effects, in vivo fate, and tumor cell mutants. J Natl Cancer Inst 1987;79:1101-12.

42. Fulton RJ, Uhr JW, Vitetta ES. In vivo therapy of the BCL₁ tumor: Effect of immunotoxin valency and deglycosylation of the ricin A chain. Cancer Res 1988;48:2626-31.

43. Smyth MJ, Pietersz GA, McKenzie IF. Use of vasoactive agents to increase tumor perfusion and the antitumor efficacy of drug-monoclonal antibody conjugates. J Natl Cancer Inst 1987;79:1367-73.

44. Blakey DC, Thorpe PE. An overview of therapy with immunotoxins containing ricin or its A chain. Antibody, Immunoconjugates, and Radiopharmacology, 1988;1:1-16.

45. Vitetta ES, Krolick KA, Miyama Inaba M, et al. Immunotoxins: A new approach to cancer therapy. Science 1983;219:644-50.

46. Spitler LE. Phase I clinical trials with immunotoxins. In: Vogel CW, ed. Immunoconjugates: Antibody conjugates in radioimaging and therapy of cancer. New York: Oxford University Press, 1987:290-300.
47. Spitler LE. Clinical studies: Solid tumors. In: Frankel AE, ed. Immunotoxins. Norwell, MA: Kluwer Academic Publishers, 1988:493-515.
48. Weiner LM, O'Dwyer J, Kitson J, et al. Phase I evaluation of an anti-breast carcinoma monoclonal antibody 260F9-recombinant ricin A chain immunoconjugate. Cancer Res 1989;49:4062-7.
49. Laurent G, Kuhlein E, Casellas P, et al. Determination of sensitivity of fresh leukemia cells to immunotoxins. Cancer Res 1986;46:2289-94.
50. Parkinson DR. Interleukin-2 in cancer therapy. In: Seminars in oncology. New York: Grune & Stratton, Inc. 1988:10-26.
51. Rosenberg SA, Lotze MT. Cancer immunotherapy using interleukin-2 and interleukin-2-activated lymphocytes. Ann Rev Immunol 1986; 4:681-709.
52. Henslee PJ, Byers VS, Jennings CD, et al. A new approach to the prevention of graft-versus-host disease using XomaZyme-H65 following histo-incompatible partially T-depleted marrow grafts. Transplant Proc 1989;21:3004-7.
53. Kernan NA, Byers VS, Scannon PJ, et al. Treatment of steroid-resistant acute graft vs host disease by in vivo administration of an anti-T-cell ricin A chain immunotoxin. JAMA 1988;259:3145-9.
54. Byers VS, Caperton E, Ackerman S, et al. Modification of the immune system in patients with rheumatoid arthritis treated with anti-CD5 ricin A chain immunotoxin. FASEB J 1989;3:A1122.
55. Vitetta ES, Stone M, Amlot P, et al. A phase I immunotoxin trial in patients with B cell lymphoma. Cancer Res, (In Press).

In: Sacher RA, Brubaker DB, Kasprisin DO and McCarthy LJ, eds.
Cellular and Humoral Immunotherapy and Apheresis
Arlington, VA: American Association of Blood Banks, 1991

5

The Human Immune Response: Cellular Aspects of Molecular Recognition and Immunoregulation

David L. Nelson, MD, and Carole C. Kurman, BS

I N THE PAST 20 YEARS, vast advances have been made toward understanding the human immune response. Progress that began with the
first morphologic definition of distinct lineages of lymphocytes has
culminated in research in which it is commonplace to molecularly clone
the genes involved in the immune response. In part, these advances have
been the result of the development of hybridoma-derived monoclonal
antibody techniques,[1] recent developments in molecular gene-cloning
technology[2] and the combination of these approaches.[3] This chapter will
focus on the central role played by T cells in the immune response (Fig
5-1), the cell surface molecules employed by immune T cells in the antigen
recognition process, the biochemical consequences of antigen recognition
and the nature and function of a series of soluble mediators that play
critical roles in the maturation and differentiation of the immune response. A better understanding of these events is likely to lead to more
effective strategies for manipulating the immune response in disease
states.

The recognition of antigen by T cells can be separated into the stages
of adhesion, antigen recognition, activation and the elaboration of lymphokines (Fig 5-2). In large part, our understanding of these events has
been the result of efficient methods for the in vitro culture of human
lymphocytes and the production of hybridoma-derived monoclonal antibodies against lymphocyte cell membrane molecules,[4] which led to the
classification of many cell surface molecules into clusters of differentia-

David L. Nelson, MD, Chief, and Carole C. Kurman, BS, Senior Research Associate,
Immunophysiology Section, Metabolism Branch, National Cancer Institute, Bethesda,
Maryland

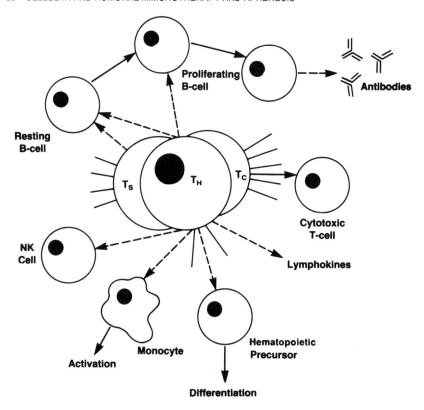

Figure 5-1. The thymus-derived T cell plays a central role in the immune response.

tion (CDs)[5] and provided both a method to study their function and a method for protein purification, sequence analysis and subsequent molecular cloning of the relevant structural genes.

Molecular Recognition and Regulation

Adhesion

Two distinct, antigen-independent adhesion pathways between T cells and antigen-presenting cells/target cells (APC/TC) have been described.[6,7] The first is mediated by the binding of the CD2 molecule (LFA-2, sheep erythrocyte receptor) on T cells to LFA-3 molecules on APC/TC, which are cation independent and temperature insensitive. The second pathway consists of the binding of LFA-1 on T cells to the ICAM-1 molecules on APC/TC, which are cation dependent and temperature sensitive. The genes

STAGES OF CELLULAR INTERACTIONS LEADING TO
T-CELL ACTIVATION

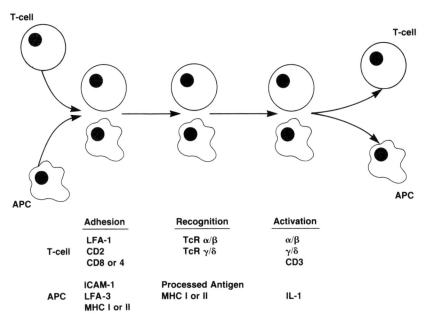

	Adhesion	Recognition	Activation
T-cell	LFA-1 CD2 CD8 or 4	TcR α/β TcR γ/δ	α/β γ/δ CD3
APC	ICAM-1 LFA-3 MHC I or II	Processed Antigen MHC I or II	IL-1

Figure 5-2. Stages of T lymphocyte antigen recognition and the cell surface molecules involved on both the T cell and the antigen-presenting cell.

encoding the CD2 molecule (LFA-2), the beta subunit of the heterodimeric LFA-1 molecule and ICAM-1 have been cloned.[3,8,9] The CD2 molecule exists as a 50-kDa cell-surface monomer and is a member of the immunoglobulin supergene family.[10] The LFA-1 antigen, a heterodimer consisting of an alpha chain of 180 kDa and a beta chain of 95 kDa, belongs to the integrin family of cell surface receptors, binding fibronectin, vitronectin and von Willebrand factor.[8] The ICAM-1 molecule has a molecular weight of 90-118 kDa and is similar to the immunoglobulin supergene family and the neural cell adhesion molecule N-CAM.[9] In addition, CD2 shows roughly the same homology to N-CAM as does ICAM-1; however, ICAM-1 and CD2 are only weakly related. These adhesive interactions apply to helper cell/APC interactions, cytotoxic T cell/target cell interactions and the binding of lymphocytes to thymic epithelium.[11] This latter observation, coupled with the finding that certain pairs of anti-CD2 antibodies alone can stimulate T-cell proliferation and maturation, have suggested an alternative antigen-independent pathway for T-cell activation,[12] which may trigger the development of the T-cell antigen receptor repertoire.

Antigen Recognition

The next stage of T-cell activation, antigen recognition, is difficult to separate from adhesion. However, additional sets of cell surface molecules are called into play. At some time during adhesion, or shortly thereafter, the products of the major histocompatibility complex (MHC) on APC/TC become important in the presentation of exogenous antigen to specific antigen receptors on the surface of immune T cells.[13,14] In humans, these polymorphic MHC antigens, located on chromosome 6, can be divided into two separate regions. The products of one region, Class I MHC molecules, consist of an integral membrane glycoprotein alpha chain with a molecular weight of 45 kDa, which is noncovalently associated with a smaller invariant β_2-microglobulin glycoprotein of 11.6 kDa, encoded by a gene on chromosome 15. The products of the second region, Class II MHC molecules, consist of two noncovalently associated glycoproteins with a heavier alpha chain of 34 kDa and a smaller beta chain of 28 kDa.

Exogenous antigens are recognized by T cells in association with the polymorphic regions of these MHC molecules. Class I and Class II molecules as well as β_2-microglobulin are all members of the immunoglobulin supergene family.[10] The variable regions of these molecules are thought to be important in antigen binding and presentation to T cells. The crystal structure of a human Class I MHC antigen was recently obtained and was found to have a pocket or groove in which "processed" exogenous antigen (and perhaps some "self" molecules) would be located[15] and presumably viewed by T cells. In general, T cells do not recognize native exogenous antigen. Foreign exogenous antigens are partially degraded in acidic endocytic vesicles prior to their association with MHC antigens, and distinct pathways for exogenous as compared to endogenously synthesized antigens may determine the association of processed antigen with either Class I or Class II MHC antigens prior to their appearance on cell surfaces.[16]

The responding T cells must have cell surface molecules (T-cell receptors) that are specifically capable of binding antigen. The vast majority of T cells utilize a heterodimeric, disulfide-linked 90-kDa antigen recognition structure consisting of a 51-kDa alpha chain and a 43-kDa beta chain. These integral membrane glycoprotein chains are encoded by genes located on separate chromosomes: chromosome 14q11 for the alpha chain, and chromosome 7q32 for the beta chain. Both are members of the immunoglobulin supergene family,[10] with alpha containing variable, joining and constant region exons, and beta containing variable, diversity, joining and constant region genes.[17] These genetic elements undergo rearrangements to produce alpha and beta gene products with variable regions and constant domains.

More recently, T cells expressing alternative T-cell antigen receptor disulfide-linked heterodimers consisting of gamma and delta chains have been described.[18,19] The size of these chains is more variable, with the gamma chain ranging from 40-55 kDa and the delta chain being 31-40 kDa. The gamma chain locus is on the short arm of chromosome 7 at 7p15, and the delta chain locus is contained within the alpha gene locus at 14q11. The gamma locus contains variable, joining and constant regions whereas the delta chain, like the beta chain, consists of variable, diversity, joining and constant region genes. Diversity in the T-cell antigen receptor protein molecules is generated by the shuffling of variable, diversity (when present), joining and constant region loci in various combinations.

Two other molecular species on the surface of T cells are involved in this antigen recognition process. The CD4 and CD8 molecules, expressed on largely nonoverlapping subsets of mature T cells, appear to play a role in which class of MHC molecules the T cells are capable of recognizing. Thus CD4+ T cells recognize antigen in the context of Class II MHC molecules, whereas CD8+ T cells recognize antigen in association with Class I MHC molecules. Both CD4 and CD8 molecules are members of the immunoglobulin supergene family,[10] and the genes encoding these molecules have been cloned.[20,21] CD4 is a 60- to 62-kDa glycoprotein expressed on the cell surface as a monomer, and CD8 is a 30- to 32-kDa glycoprotein expressed as a disulfide-linked multimer.[22] It is not known whether the CD4 and CD8 molecules bind to the same Class I and Class II MHC molecules containing processed antigen to which the T-cell antigen receptor binds, or to other MHC molecules. The binding of the T-cell antigen receptor and CD4 and CD8 molecules on the T cell surface to antigen bound to MHC Class I and II antigens on APC/TC triggers a series of biochemical sequences that result in the growth and maturation of antigen-specific T cells and the elaboration of a variety of soluble factors, as well as biochemical changes in the APC/TC.

Activation

In addition to the molecules already engaged in the T-cell/APC/TC interaction, at least two additional sets of molecules are involved in the subsequent activation of T cells. The first series of molecules, the CD3 complex, consists of at least four and perhaps as many as six distinct molecules. Four of the genes—the gamma, delta, epsilon and zeta—have been cloned. This complex is intimately associated with the T-cell antigen receptor (TcR) heterodimers (alpha/beta or gamma/delta). CD3 gamma and CD3 delta are glycoproteins of 25 and 20 kDa, respectively, whereas CD3 epsilon is nonglycosylated and has a molecular weight of 20 kDa. These three genes are clearly related and probably arose from a common ancestor. CD3 delta and epsilon map close to each other on human chromosome 11 at 11q23 and are oriented in head to tail fashion no more than two kilobases apart. Association within the TcR/CD3 complex may be between negatively charged amino acids in the transmembrane region of CD3 gamma and delta and positively charged amino acids in the transmembrane of the T-cell antigen receptor alpha/beta or gamma/delta chains. Only recently has the CD3 zeta molecule been cloned. It is an approximately 16-kDa molecule, expressed as a disulfide-linked homodimer, and is unrelated to the other CD3 molecules. The molecule has a short extracellular domain and a long intracytoplasmic tail with numerous tyrosines, which are phosphorylated following cellular activation. The CD3 zeta molecule also contains a consensus nucleotide binding site. This molecule seems a likely candidate for signal transduction to the cytoplasm following cellular activation via TcR/CD3. The gene encoding CD3 zeta is located on chromosome 1.

The likely composition of the TcR/CD3 complex is one molecule each of CD3 gamma, delta, epsilon, TcR alpha (or gamma) and TcR beta (or delta), and two molecules of CD3 zeta. The signal-transducing biochemical processes resulting from T-cell activation via the TcR/CD3 complex appear similar to those seen in many cell types. Central to this process is the hydrolysis of membrane inositol phospholipid and the generation of second messengers within the cell.[23] T-cell perturbation through the TcR/CD3 complex leads to the activation of a phosphodiesterase that hydrolyzes phospholipid phosphatidylinositol bisphosphate to generate inositol triphosphate (IP3) and diacylglycerol. Subsequently, IP3 increases release of Ca^{2++} from intracellular stores, thereby increasing the concentration of free intracellular Ca^{2++}. This process may stimulate Ca^{2++}-dependent protein kinases, resulting in protein phosphorylation. IP3 is subsequently converted to inositol bisphosphate, inositol phosphate and inositol, which can reenter the cell membrane. Diacylglycerol activates the enzyme protein kinase C, in part by increasing its affinity for Ca^{2++}, and results in a translocation of the enzyme from the cytosol to the cell membrane. The enzyme subsequently catalyzes the phosphorylation of numerous proteins at seryl and threonyl residues, using adenosine triphosphate as a phosphate donor. By an as yet undefined mechanism, these second messengers signal the nucleus, inducing a series of transcriptional events either directly or indirectly influencing gene expression.

This activation process for T cells also has direct consequences for the activation of APC. It induces the synthesis and release of a cytokine termed interleukin-1 (IL-1), which has diverse metabolic properties.[24] Two biochemically distinct but structurally related IL-1 molecules have been cloned: IL-1 beta and IL-1 alpha. These two interleukins share only small stretches (26%) of amino acid homology. Each is coded by separate genes on chromosome 2. Both forms are unique in that they are initially translated as precursor polypeptides (31 kDa), and despite the fact that IL-1 is found as a secreted product, neither contains a signal cleavage sequence. The generation of the mature peptide (17 kDa) and smaller peptides occurs by serine protease cleavage; a considerable amount of IL-1 remains cell-associated as part of the cell membrane. The 31-kDa IL-1 precursor and a 22-kDa form are membrane bound. Membrane-bound IL-1 is biologically active and may account for a significant part of the immunostimulatory effects of IL-1. IL-1 stimulates the production of a variety of lymphokines by activated T cells, including IL-2, the interferons, IL-3 and other bone marrow colony-stimulating factors, and IL-6. Particular attention has focused on the role of IL-1 in T-cell responses. With T-cell lines, pM concentrations of IL-1 induce the transcription, synthesis and secretion of IL-2 as well as the expression of IL-2 receptors. These responses to IL-1 are greatly enhanced (10- to 100-fold) by agents that raise cytosolic calcium and activate protein kinase C.

Secretion of
Soluble Molecules

These events described above trigger the synthesis and secretion of a variety of soluble factors by activated T cells. Because many of these soluble factors have effects on other leukocytes, they have been termed interleukins. Some of these lymphokines influence T-cell responses, whereas others influence cells of the B-cell series as well as granulocytes and cells of several primitive hematopoietic lineages. In order to clonally expand and promptly respond to antigen, T cells must divide and differentiate.

One lymphokine playing a major role in this process is IL-2. IL-2, produced by activated T cells, stimulates the proliferation and effector function of activated T cells, natural killer (NK) cells and cytotoxic T cells. IL-2 directly affects B cells and macrophages and also induces/enhances production of other cytokines, such as IL-3, IL-4, colony-stimulating factors and interferons.[25,26] It appears to play a central role in the regulation of immune function and hematopoietic cell growth and differentiation. IL-2 is a molecule of 14.5-17 kDa; the size range is due to differential glycosylation.

Both major T-cell subsets (CD4+ and CD8+) are capable of producing IL-2. A cloned cDNA for human IL-2 has been obtained. The IL-2 gene is located on chromosome 4 at 4q26-28. Although IL-2 does not enhance its own production, it has been shown to enhance T-cell production of granulocyte-monocyte colony-stimulating factor (GM-CSF) and interferon-γ. The binding of IL-2 to its receptor on T cells will induce further expression of IL-2 receptors. IL-2 will also induce B-cell proliferation and maturation. To exert its effect, IL-2 must interact with specific high-affinity membrane receptors for IL-2. These receptors are expressed not on resting cells but on activated T cells, B cells[27] and monocytes.[28] IL-2 receptors are composed of at least two molecules, the p55 Tac peptide and a 75-kDa molecule.[29] Additional evidence has been presented for a 95-kDa component of the receptor.[30] In addition to being a component of the cellular high-affinity receptor for IL-2, soluble Tac protein of low affinity is released from activated T cells, B cells and monocytes.[31]

Two other factors produced by activated T cells have effects on multiple lineages of hematopoietic cells: GM-CSF and multi-colony-stimulating factor (IL-3). These factors are so named because of their capacity to stimulate colonies in soft agar. GM-CSF, which has a molecular weight of 14-35 kDa, stimulates cells of neutrophile, monocyte, eosinophile, erythroid and megakaryocyte lineages. IL-3 has a molecular weight of 14-28 kDa and also stimulates cells of the same lineages. The size heterogeneity of IL-3 is due to glycosylation, with carbohydrate comprising 50% of some molecules. These factors appear to have no effect on T cells or B cells. Computer analysis of the gene sequences of GM-CSF and human IL-3 failed to reveal any significant sequence homology despite some common structural features and the fact that both are expressed in activated T cells. It is interesting that both the human GM-CSF and IL-3 genes have been mapped to the same band on the long arm of chromosome 5 in a region known to contain the genes for macrophage colony-stimulating factor and its receptor, as well as the genes for several other growth factors and growth factor receptors.[32]

Activated T cells also secrete lymphokines that have major effects on B-cell proliferation and differentiation into immunoglobulin-secreting plasma cells. Three such factors are IL-4, IL-5 and IL-6. IL-4 has the property of inducing the proliferation of activated B cells (B-cell growth factor). However, this lymphokine and IL-5 must both be considered as multifunctional molecules. They affect the development of several cell lineages (IL-4 affects B cells, T cells, mast cells and macrophages) and can affect different stages of the same lineage (IL-4 will act on both resting and activated B cells). IL-4 and IL-5 are molecules of 14.1 and 12.3 kDa, respectively, and both share limited but significant homology with GM-CSF and interferon-γ, suggesting a remote phylogenetic relationship of these cytokines.[33] The gene for IL-5 is located on chromosome 5. IL-4 increases the expression of Class II MHC molecules and Fc receptors for IgE on the surface of resting B cells, induces DNA synthesis by IL-2-dependent T-cell lines, may induce the growth of early lymphoid precursors in bone marrow (pro-T cells and pro-pre-B cells) and induces the growth of mast cells. IL-5 causes the differentiation of activated B cells into immunoglobulin-secreting cells, increases synthesis of the secretory form of IgM, upregulates IL-2 receptor expression on B cells, induces cytotoxic T cells and causes eosinophile differentiation.

IL-6 and interferon-β_2 are identical and can be produced by a variety of cell types both constitutively and upon stimulation. IL-6 has a number of functions, including antiviral activity, growth inhibition of fibroblasts, stimulation of growth of human B cells,[34] stimulation of differentiation of proliferating B cells into plasma cells and the induction of acute phase proteins in hepatocytes. Mature IL-6 is a molecule of 26 kDa that lacks strong homology to IL-1, IL-2, γ-interferon, GM-CSF or IL-4. The IL-6 gene is located on chromosome 7. IL-1 is a very efficient inducer of IL-6 secretion by activated T cells.

Although it is not the product of activated T cells, the cytokine IL-7 affects the development of T and B cells. This cytokine is constitutively produced by thymic and bone marrow stromal cells. IL-7, a 25-kDa molecule, stimulates the proliferation of pre-B cells, and the proliferation and differentiation of thymocytes and mature T cells. The gene encoding IL-7 has been cloned; it resides on chromosome 8 at 8q12q13. IL-7 most likely encodes a protein molecule of the "helix loop helix" class of DNA binding proteins.

γ-interferon, a molecule of 20-25 kDa, is encoded by a gene on chromosome 12 and produced by activated T cells and NK cells. Interferon-γ increases the proliferation and differentiation of activated B cells, synergizes with IL-2 for the proliferation and differentiation of activated B cells, synergizes with IL-4 for the proliferation of activated B cells and antagonizes the IL-4-induced B-cell expression of FcR epsilon and IgE secretion. It also causes increased NK effector activity, increased Fc IgG receptor expression and tumoricidal activity by monocytes and enhances MHC Class II expression on endothelial cells and fibroblasts.

Two unique subsets of T cells, cytotoxic T cells and suppressor T cells, have been associated with the secretion of classes of less well-characterized soluble factors. Although intimate contact is required between the cytotoxic effector T cell and the target cell being lysed, most available data support the notion that the lytic event is mediated by a soluble factor(s) secreted by cytotoxic T cells. Various factors are being considered as candidates, including molecules capable of forming pores or channels in target cell membranes (such as cytolysin and the polyperforins) and non-pore-forming molecules, including tumor necrosis factor (TNF alpha), lymphotoxin (TNF beta), the interferons and both IL-1 alpha and beta.[35] Suppressor cells also secrete a series of molecules, including a 10- to 15-kDa soluble immune response suppressor, which must be oxidized in monocytes prior to gaining activity. Soluble immune suppressor substance-B and -T, which are also secreted by suppressor cells, show relative specificity for suppression of B- and T-cell responses, respectively.[36]

Conclusion

Recent advances in cellular and molecular immunology have provided the foundation for understanding the molecular basis of the immune response. These technologies have created recombinant DNA-derived molecules that can be purified and functionally isolated. These molecules and their receptors can now be the targets of strategies for manipulating the immune response in certain disease states. The next level of understanding will be at the level of protein/DNA interactions that control the transcription and translation of these genes. In addition to certain structural similarities among the genes for these molecules, several of these genes (GM-CSF, IL-2, IL-4, IL-5, interferon-γ and granulocyte colony-stimulating factor) share nucleotide sequence motifs in their 5' ends; this may play a role in the regulation of the expression of these genes.[37] The genes encoding the proteins that bind these motifs and their regulatory elements will extend this knowledge even further and will provide new insights and strategies for understanding and manipulating the human immune response.

References

1. Köhler G, Milstein C. Continuous cultures of fused cells secreting antibody of predefined specificity. Nature 1975;256:495-7.
2. Maniatis T, Fritsch EF, Sambrook J, eds. Molecular cloning: A Laboratory manual. Cold Spring Harbor: Cold Spring Harbor Press, 1982.
3. Seed B, Aruffo A. Molecular cloning of the CD2 antigen, the T-cell erythrocyte receptor, by a rapid immunoselection procedure. Proc Natl Acad Sci USA 1987;84:3365.
4. McMichael AJ, Pilch JR, Galfrie G, et al. A human thymocyte antigen defined by a hybrid myeloma monoclonal antibody. Eur J Immunol 1979;9:205-10.
5. McMichael A, Beverley TCL, Cobbold S, eds. Leukocyte typing III. Oxford: Oxford University Press, 1987.
6. Shaw S, Ginther Luce GE, Quinones R, et al. Two antigen-independent adhesion pathways used by human cytotoxic T-cell clones. Nature 1986;323:262-4.
7. Makgoba MW, Sanders ME, Ginther Luce GE, et al. ICAM-1 a ligand for LFA-1 dependent adhesion of B, T, and myeloid cells. Nature 1988;331:86-8.
8. Kishimoto TK, O'Connor K, Lee A, et al. Cloning of the beta subunit of the leukocyte adhesion proteins: Homology to an extracellular matrix receptor defines a novel supergene family. Cell 1987;48:681-90.
9. Simmons D, Makgoba MW, Seed B. ICAM, an adhesion ligand of LFA-1, is homologous to the neural cell adhesion molecule NCAM. Nature 1988;331:624-7.
10. Hood L, Kronenberg M, Hunkapiller T. T cell antigen receptors and the immunoglobulin supergene family. Cell 1985;40:225-9.
11. Vollger LW, Tuck DT, Springer TA, et al. Thymocyte binding to human thymic epithelial cells is inhibited by monoclonal antibodies to CD-2 and LFA-3 antigens. J Immunol 1987;138:358.
12. Meuer SC, Hussey RE, Fabbi M, et al. An alternative pathway of T cell activation: A functional role for the 50 kd T11 sheep erythrocyte receptor protein. Cell 1984;36:897-906.
13. Zinkernagel RM, Doherty PC. Restriction of in vitro T-cell mediated cytotoxicity in lymphocytic choriomeningitis within a syngeneic or semiallogeneic system. Nature 1974;248:701-2.

14. Shearer GM, Rehn TG, Garbarino CA. Cell mediated lympholysis of trinitrophenyl-modified cell surface components controlled by the H-2K and H-2D serological regions of the murine major histocompatibility complex. J Exp Med 1975;141:1438-64.

15. Bjorkman PJ, Saper MA, Samraoui B, et al. Structure of the human class I histocompatibility antigen, HLA-A2. Nature 1987;329:506-12.

16. Braciale TJ, Morrison LA, Sweetser MT, et al. Antigen presentation pathways to class I and class II MHC-restricted T lymphocytes. Immunol Rev 1987;98:95-114.

17. Toyonaga B, Mak TW. Genes of the T-cell antigen receptor in normal and malignant T-cells. Annu Rev Immunol 1987;5:585-620.

18. Brenner MB, McLean J, Dialynas DP, et al. Identification of a putative second T-cell receptor. Nature 1986;322:145-9.

19. Bank I, DePinho RA, Brenner MB, et al. A functional T3 molecule associated with a novel heterodimer on the surface of immature human thymocytes. Nature 1986;322:179-81.

20. Madden PJ, Littman DR, Godfrey M, et al. The isolation and nucleotide sequence of a cDNA encoding the T cell surface protein T4: A new member of the immunoglobulin gene family. Cell 1985;42:93-104.

21. Sukhatme VP, Sizer KC, Vollmer AC, et al. The T cell differentiation antigen Leu-2/T8 is homologous to immunoglobulin and T cell receptor variable regions. Cell 1985;40:591-7.

22. Littman DR. The structure of the CD4 and CD8 genes. Annu Rev Immunol 1987;5:561-84.

23. Weiss A, Imboden J, Hardy K, et al. The role of the T3/antigen receptor complex in T-cell activation. Annu Rev Immunol 1986;4:593-619.

24. Dinarello CA. Biology of interleukin-1. FASEB J 1988;2:108-15.

25. Mertelsmann R, Welte K. Human interleukin 2: Molecular biology, physiology and clinical possibilities. Immunobiology 1986;172:400-19.

26. Farrar JJ, Benjamin WR, Hilfiker ML, et al. The biochemistry, biology, and role of interleukin 2 in the induction of cytotoxic T cell and antibody-forming B cell responses. Immunol Rev 1982;63:129-66.

27. Waldmann TA, Goldman CK, Robb RJ, et al. Expression of interleukin 2 receptors on activated human B cells. J Exp Med 1984;160:1450-66.

28. Holter W, Goldman CK, Casabo L, et al. Expression of functional IL 2 receptors by lipopolysaccharide and interferon-gamma stimulated human monocytes. J Immunol 1987;138:2917-22.

29. Waldmann TA. The role of the multichain IL-2 receptor complex in the control of normal and malignant T-cell proliferation. Environ Health Perspect 1987;75:11-5.

30. Szollosi J, Damjanovich S, Goldman CK, et al. Flow cytometric resonance energy transfer measurements support the association of a 95-kDa peptide termed T27 with the 55-kDa2 Tac peptide. Proc Natl Acad Sci USA 1987;84:7246-50.

31. Nelson DL, Wagner DK, Marcon L, et al. An analysis of soluble interleukin-2 receptors in human neoplastic disorders. In: Albertini A, Lenfant C, Paoletti R, eds. Biotechnology in clinical medicine. New York: Raven Press, 1987:277-86.

32. Clark SC, Kamen R. The human hematopoietic colony stimulating factors. Science 1987;236:1229-37.

33. Sideras P, Noma T, Honjo T. Structure and function of interleukin 4 and 5. Immunol Rev 1988;102:189-212.

34. Tosato G, Seamon KB, Goldman ND, et al. Monocyte-derived human B-cell growth factor identified as interferon-Beta2 (BSF-2, IL-6). Science 1988;239:502-4.

35. Koren HS, Goldfarb R, Henkart P, et al. Proposal for classification of leukocyte-associated cytolytic molecules. J Leukoc Biol 1987;41:447-9.

36. Rich RR, ElMasry MN, Fox EJ. Human suppressor T-cells: Induction, differentiation, and regulatory functions. Hum Immunol 1986;17: 369-87.

37. Yokota T, Arai N, deVries J, et al. Molecular biology of interleukin 4 and interleukin 5 genes and biology of their products that stimulate B cells, T cells and hemopoietic cells. Immunol Rev 1988;102:137-87.

In: Sacher RA, Brubaker DB, Kasprisin DO and McCarthy LJ, eds.
Cellular and Humoral Immunotherapy and Apheresis
Arlington, VA: American Association of Blood Banks, 1991

6

Peripheral Blood Stem Cell Collection and Use

Larry C. Lasky, MD

I N MARROW TRANSPLANTATION, THE infused marrow provides a source of hematopoietic progenitors that eventually grow into mature blood cells. Since hematopoietic progenitor cells circulate in the blood, cells isolated from the circulation may be used as an alternative to marrow. This may be possible and desirable in certain situations such as marrow involvement with malignancy, damage to the posterior iliac crests (where marrow is generally collected) by radiation or infection, or inability to undergo general anesthesia for marrow harvest. This may also be more acceptable to allogeneic donors than procurement of progenitor cells from the bone marrow. There may be other advantages over the use of marrow.

Early Work

Animal Studies

Cross-circulation studies in animals, in which animals irradiated to destroy their marrow were connected by arteriovenous anastomosis to nonirradiated ones, showed that the cells capable of repopulating both the marrow and the immunologic system were in the circulation.[1,2] Further studies showed that mononuclear leukocytes collected from canine blood could be used in both autologous and allogeneic settings to rescue dogs from marrow-ablative radio/chemotherapy.[3-5]

Larry C. Lasky, MD, Associate Director, Memorial Blood Center of Minneapolis, Minneapolis, Minnesota

In Vitro Studies

As a prelude to actual use of peripheral blood stem cells (PBSCs) as a source of hematopoietic progenitors for transplantation, numerous studies were carried out in vitro. The characteristics of blood- vs marrow-derived hematopoietic progenitors were examined using semisolid clonogenic assays and long-term liquid culture. While committed myeloid [granulocyte-macrophage colony-forming units (CFU-GM)] and erythroid [erythrocyte burst-forming units (BFU-E)] progenitors are found in the circulation of hematopoietically normal individuals, certain differences between progenitors from blood and marrow do exist. The more committed erythroid progenitor [erythrocyte colony-forming units (CFU-E)] cannot be cultured from blood, and multipotent progenitors (CFU-MIX or CFU-GEMM) from blood have both less self-renewal capability and less tendency to differentiate in vitro into megakaryocytes.[6,7] Blood-derived CFU-GM colonies more often consist of eosinophils than colonies grown from marrow.[8] The size and density of progenitors from blood and marrow appear to be similar.[9] Marrow (but not peripheral blood) derived progenitor populations can produce a supportive adherent layer in long-term culture.[10]

Human Preclinical Studies

Several related studies laid the background for actual use of peripheral-blood-derived progenitors as cellular support in humans. When chronic myelogenous leukemia (CML) cells were used to treat or prevent infection in non-CML patients, occasional patients experienced engraftment of the malignant cells, as demonstrated by chromosome studies.[11] Autologous CML peripheral blood cells rescued patients from marrow-ablative radio/chemotherapy. Generally, chronic phase CML rather than normal hematopoiesis was established. When cells collected during chronic phase CML were used in blast crisis, survival may have been prolonged in some patients.[12] Rarely, normal hematopoiesis was reestablished.[13]

Buffy coat cells were used as a supplement to marrow from normal donors in transplantation of aplastic anemia patients at risk for rejection. These cells successfully lowered the incidence of rejection, but caused a marked increase in the incidence of graft-vs-host disease (GVHD).[14]

Large numbers of progenitors can be isolated from subjects in the course of routine platelet/leukocyte apheresis collections, and during collections specifically designed to collect progenitors, which are in the mononuclear (lymphocyte plus monocyte) fraction of the white cells.[15,16] Extending the collection to as long as 3 hours does not seem to diminish the number of committed progenitors collected or in the circulation.[17] Progenitors can be frozen successfully using techniques established for marrow, eg, 10% dimethylsulfoxide (DMSO), controlled-rate freezing and storage in the liquid phase of liquid nitrogen.[15]

Methods of Collection

Machines

Several types of apheresis machines have been used to collect PBSCs for clinical use. A procedure optimized to collect monocytes and/or lymphocytes (the so-called "mononuclear cells") affords the best yield of committed hematopoietic cells. The instrument most often reported has been the Fenwal CS3000 (Baxter Healthcare Corporation, Deerfield, IL), a computer-controlled, continuous flow machine. Methods developed for the collection of lymphocytes for production of lymphokine-activated killer (LAK) cells work well. An increased centrifuge speed of 1400 RPM increases mononuclear cell yield while lowering neutrophil collection.[15] The latter is important, since the freeze-thaw methods used for PBSC collection cause lysis of neutrophils and, if too many are collected, subsequent processing before cryopreservation is needed. Unfortunately, procedures optimized for collection of mononuclear cells also tend to collect platelets because of their similarity in density. Thus, when using these procedures on the CS3000, it is sometimes necessary to perform a low-speed centrifugation (a "soft spin") during the PBSC collection to separate and return a portion of the collected platelets. This can be done in the CS3000 itself. Some investigators use hydroxyethyl starch during the procedure,[18] although most do not. Additional machines that have been used include the discontinued AMINCO Celltrifuge (American Instrument Company, Silver Spring, MD),[19] the Haemonetics Model 30 (Haemonetics Corporation, Braintree, MA),[20,21] the V50 (Haemonetics Corporation, Braintree, MA)[20] and the Cobe Spectra (COBE Laboratories, Lakewood, CO).

Techniques

Processing Before Cryopreservation

If multiple collections are needed, the volume to be infused can be large. Red cells and granulocytes are lysed by the freeze-thaw cycle, so it is helpful to minimize the content of these in the material eventually infused. A simple centrifugation can be used to reduce the volume before cryopreservation. To remove the majority of the red cells, a buffy coat can be made. To remove red cells and neutrophils, some have performed a Ficoll-diatrizoate or Percoll discontinuous density gradient centrifugation prior to freezing.[22,23] With procedures designed to collect only mononuclear cells and to reject red cells and granulocytes, such postcollection removal of red cells is not necessary.

Malignant Cell Contamination

One possible advantage of the use of PBSCs over marrow is in cases where the marrow is involved with malignancy, as PBSCs have less malignant cell contamination than marrow. In Hodgkin's disease, almost all disease spread can be attributed to travel in the lymphatics rather than the blood. In one study of PBSC rescue in Hodgkin's disease, relapse or recurrent disease only occurred at the site of previous disease, supporting the belief that malignant cells capable of forming metastases do not circulate.[24] In 28 tested PBSC collections from six patients (five with Stage III or IV neuroblastoma and one with Wilm's tumor), specific stains for neoplastic cells with a sensitivity of one cell in 10^5 only detected such cells in two collections from one patient.[25] To et al[26] could not detect residual leukemia in PBSC harvested in very early remission of acute nonlymphocytic leukemia (ANLL) patients.

Preservation

Cryopreservation is performed as for autologous marrow. The most common approach is to use a final concentration of 10% DMSO and controlled-rate freezing. The concentrate is stored in the liquid phase of liquid nitrogen. Storage can be in tubes or bags.[27] Since all or a large part of an apheresis collection can be stored in one to three bags, this method is much more convenient. In centers where tubes are used (and in some where bags are used) cells are thawed, diluted with a large volume of media (usually 10 times the volume of the frozen cell concentrate), washed, pooled and infused into the patient. In the majority of centers, PBSC preparations, similar to marrow preparations, are thawed in a 37-40 C waterbath and infused directly into the patient. In this case, the patient's blood accomplishes the dilution of the DMSO solution that is achieved manually in the thaw-wash-pool method. Cell clumping, which is a frequent problem during the in vitro manipulation of cryopreserved PBSCs and marrow, is generally avoided by the direct infusion method. Also, postthaw exposure to DMSO, which is toxic to progenitor cells in the liquid state, is minimized.

An alternative approach to cryopreservation has been reported in which a combination of DMSO and hydroxyethyl starch are used along with freezing in a mechanical freezer at –80 C, and storage at –80 C. The single study in which this has been used with PBSC described marked delay in platelet engraftment, and this modified freezing procedure must be considered as a possible explanation.[21,28,29]

Dose

The dose of PBSC used in different studies varies considerably. The number of cells used depends to some degree on the circumstances of the harvest and on the preparative regimen that will precede the PBSC infusion. If PBSC collection is being performed during rebound following chemotherapy, fewer cells will be needed since the number of at least committed progenitors per cell collected will be higher. In these circumstances, as few as $2\text{-}3 \times 10^8$ nucleated cells per kg of patient mass have been used.[19,30] Otherwise, if collections have been performed without some method of increasing circulating progenitor numbers, a dose of $6\text{-}8 \times 10^8$ cells per kg has been used. If the preparative regimen is not myeloablative, and the PBSC infusion is meant to merely shorten the period of severe aplasia, fewer cells may be required than when a permanently myeloablative treatment is used.

The number of progenitors (as measured by clonogenic assay) needed to enhance recovery is a controversial one, as it is in the case of autologous marrow transplantation.[31] There is no current reliable assay for the cell responsible for engraftment in human marrow transplantation. Rather than assaying for this primordial undifferentiated and self-renewing cell, current assays measure the presence of colony-forming units of a more or less committed nature. A large part of the controversy arises from the nature of the assays themselves. The assays, including the most-used CFU-GM, can be performed in many ways, and different institutions use different techniques or variations of the same technique. The assays can be affected by such factors as source of colony-stimulating activity [eg, lymphocyte feeder layer, phytohemagglutinin-stimulated leukocyte-conditioned medium (PHA-LCM), recombinant GM- or G- or M-CSF, Mo-cell conditioned medium, etc], incubation conditions (eg, 20% or 5% O_2; 4%, 5% or 7.5% CO_2), other nonprogenitor cells in the population being plated (eg, monocytes can be either inhibitory or stimulatory if not removed before plating, depending on culture conditions) and other culture ingredients (eg, lot number of fetal calf serum; presence, type and amount of steroids and reducing agents used; etc). In published studies, these factors are often not explicitly stated and, when they are, they vary considerably. Moreover, only rarely are reference ranges provided so that the reader can evaluate the numbers given in light of some standard.

Within one institution, however, if a consistent culture technique is used, the results may be useful. One group has proposed a level of CFU-GM infused below which recovery is delayed or temporary in their institution. This level in their experience appears to be 50×10^4 CFU-GM per kg. They have examined the use of the less committed CFU-GEMM or CFU-MIX, but have found that it rises in concert with the CFU-GM level during cyclic chemotherapy rebound, and hence is no better a predictor of hematopoietic recovery.[32,33] In a study of the available literature, these investigators found that a dose above 30×10^4 CFU-GM per kg afforded rapid and prolonged engraftment. Another group has proposed 15×10^4 CFU-GM per kg as the cutoff, based on 72 PBSC rescues performed in France.[34] However, several groups have reported successful enduring hematopoietic recoveries using considerably lower doses of CFU-GM, as much as one to two orders of magnitude lower.[35,36]

Additional culture techniques that more closely represent the repopulating cell may be possible in the future. Ogawa's group[37] has described an assay for marrow progenitors that produce self-renewing and differentiating blast-like cells in vitro. From their in vitro characteristics, these cells are apparently much closer in the differentiation pathway to the primordial marrow repopulating cell than progenitors measured in the assays described above. The problem with the current application of this assay in evaluation of PBSC populations is that even in marrow these cells are extremely rare, and they have yet to be cultured from peripheral blood other than cord blood. Douay et al[10] have examined the ability of PBSCs to establish long-term "marrow" cultures. They found they could establish long-term CFU-GM production using PBSCs in the absence of an adherent marrow stroma cell layer. This, too, may be used in the future to evaluate PBSC preparations for their marrow restoration potential.

Methods To Enhance
the Number of
Progenitor Cells Collected

Several manipulations have been shown to increase the number of committed progenitors in the circulation. Since the apheresis procedure collection efficiency for committed progenitors appears to be relatively constant, the number collected will rise as the number circulating in the subject increases. Procedures to increase the number of circulating progenitors include manipulation involving exercise, diurnal change, a previous apheresis collection and administration of endotoxin, steroids, epinephrine, adrenocorticotropic hormone, erythropoietin, GM-CSF or dextran.[38-44] The increase in circulating numbers during the circulating white cell and platelet rise following marrow-suppressive chemotherapy has been used most successfully.[45,46]

Recombinant GM-CSF has recently been described to increase the number of circulating committed progenitors, and this may be used to raise the number collected in clinical situations in the future.[44] Erythropoietin has been shown to increase the number of circulating erythroid and other committed progenitors in uremics.[43] It may be practical to use growth factors in situations in which chemotherapy cannot or should not be used to induce a rebound increase in circulating progenitors. This would be true in allogeneic PBSC transplantation.

Clinical Studies

Clinical disorders in which nonleukemic PBSCs have been used include acute leukemia, Hodgkin's and non-Hodgkin's lymphoma, and various solid tumors, including breast and small cell carcinoma of the lung. With one reported exception in the treatment of malignancy, these have been for autologous rather than allogeneic infusion.

The largest reported number of patients has been those with ANLL.[19,22,30,47-52] These patients were generally harvested in very early remission, as the number of circulating progenitors reached a peak following chemotherapy. Recovery was usually rapid and sustained, with the absolute neutrophil count reaching 500/μL on or about day 10 after infusion. Hematopoietic recovery was usually sustained, although some have reported a lowering of counts 2-3 weeks after infusion when lower numbers of committed progenitors have been infused.[53] Some controversy exists over the relapse rate, ranging from none to 75% in studies reporting patients transplanted in first remission.[49,51] Peripheral blood stem cells have also been used in a small number of cases of acute lymphoblastic leukemia. [22]

Lymphomas and solid tumors represent the next most frequently reported areas in which PBSCs have been used.[18,20,21,24,25,35,54,55] In a study by Kessinger et al,[20] in which 10 patients—six with breast cancer, three with Hodgkin's disease and one with non-Hodgkin's lymphoma—were treated using PBSCs as cellular support, eight 4-hour collections were performed in each patient using a variety of machines. Rebound after chemotherapy was not used to increase the number of circulating progenitors. Only one patient, with non-Hodgkin's lymphoma, was alive with no evidence of disease at the time of the report. Another study compared the use of PBSCs in seven Hodgkin's lymphoma patients to the use of marrow in 19 similarly treated patients.[24] This study showed that hematopoietic recovery was faster in the PBSC-treated group than in the marrow-treated group. There was a shorter hospital stay (by about 1 week) in the PBSC-treated patients, too, but this difference lacked statistical significance. In this study, five to eight 3-hour apheresis collections from each patient were performed using the Fenwal CS3000.

In a study by Stiff et al,[21] eight patients with small cell carcinoma of the lung were treated with PBSCs that were collected during the recovery phase following cyclic chemotherapy. They used the Haemonetics Model 30, performing an average of four to five 3- to 3.5-hour collections. Their PBSC patients' platelet recoveries were markedly prolonged. The delay in platelet recovery may possibly be explained by their use of an alternative cryopreservation technique.

PBSCs have been reported used in the treatment of Stage III or IV childhood neuroblastoma.[25,35,56] Children as small as 8.3 kg donated PBSCs on a Fenwal CS3000 primed with red cells and fresh frozen plasma. No difficulties were encountered in these small patients, in whom central lines were used for venous access. Hematopoietic recovery was comparable to or faster than that in similarly treated marrow-rescued patients.

The T cells present in even an HLA-identical marrow (or, presumably, PBSC preparation) are capable of producing GVHD in the recipient.[57] On the other hand, probably a certain number of T cells are necessary for engraftment of an allogeneic marrow and, again presumably, allogeneic PBSCs. Since about 80% of the mononuclear cells in peripheral blood are T cells, their elimination can be a problem. Dooley et al[58] have developed a discontinuous Percoll gradient, sheep red cell rosetting procedure that can accomplish a 20-fold reduction in the number of T cells in a PBSC collection. This was used in a single reported attempt at allogeneic transplantation using PBSCs in treating a malignancy.[59] This acute lymphoblastic leukemia patient experienced hematopoietic recovery but died on day 32 from infectious complications, and too soon to be evaluated for GVHD. If the problems can be worked out, however, the possibility of the use of PBSCs in the allogeneic setting is an attractive one, especially in unrelated donor-recipient scenarios.

Future Enhancements and Applications

Other Growth Factor Applications

GM-CSF and G-CSF and perhaps other growth factors offer potential means to significantly and safely increase the number of progenitors circulating and hence collected. It may be possible to use recombinant growth factors such as interleukin-3 or GM-CSF to treat already-collected PBSCs to expand the number of progenitors ex vivo. A third possible application of growth factors is after infusion, to speed multiplication and differentiation of infused progenitors. This has been successful after autologous marrow, and presumably will be after PBSC infusion.[60]

Combination With Marrow

Marrow reconstitution after autologous marrow infusion can be delayed considerably, but is generally durable once established. Conversely, reconstitution after PBSC infusion is relatively rapid, but can regress after a period of days to weeks in certain situations. One possible strategy to make better use of the properties of hematopoietic recovery after each form of cellular support has been infused is to combine them. This has been reported in the case of a patient with Ewing's sarcoma.[61]

Combination With IL-2/LAK Cells

Another attractive possibility is to utilize the hematopoietic progenitors in lymphocyte collections performed in the preparation of LAK cells. Although the combination of autologous marrow and LAK cells and/or interleukin-2 (IL-2) infusion has been proposed and/or reported, exploitation of the combination of PBSCs and LAK/IL-2 infusion has yet to be reported.[62-64]

Acknowledgments

The author thanks Dr. Jeffrey McCullough for inviting him to write a review on this subject for *Transfusion*, on which the present review is based.[65]

References

1. Epstein RB, Graham TC, Buckner CD, et al. Allogeneic marrow engraftment by cross circulation in lethally irradiated dogs. Blood 1966;28:692-707.
2. Storb R, Graham TC, Epstein RB, et al. Demonstration of hemopoietic stem cells in the peripheral blood of baboons by cross circulation. Blood 1977;50:537-42.
3. Abrams RA, McCormack K, Bowles C, Deisseroth AB. Cyclophosphamide treatment expands the circulating hematopoietic stem cell pool in dogs. J Clin Invest 1981;67:1392-9.
4. Körbling M, Fliedner TM, Calvo C, et al. Albumin density gradient purification of canine hemopoietic blood stem cells (HBSC): Long-term allogeneic engraftment without GVH-reaction. Exp Hematol 1979;7:277-88.
5. Zander AR, Gray KN, Hester JP, et al. Rescue by peripheral blood mononuclear cells in dogs from bone marrow failure after total-body irradiation. Transfusion 1984;24:42-5.
6. Ash RC, Detrick RA, Zanjani ED. Studies of human pluripotential hemopoietic stem cells (CFU-GEMM) in vitro. Blood 1981;58:309-16.
7. Ganser A, Elstner E, Hoelzer D. Megakaryocytic cells in mixed haemopoietic colonies (CFU-GEMM) from the peripheral blood of normal individuals. Br J Haematol 1985;59:627-33.
8. Verma DS, Spitzer G, Zander AR, et al. The myeloid progenitor cell: A parallel study of subpopulations in human marrow and peripheral blood. Exp Hematol 1980;8:32-43.
9. Lasky LC, Zanjani ED. Size and density characterization of human committed and multipotent hematopoietic progenitors. Exp Hematol 1985;13:680-4.

10. Douay L, Lefrançois G, Castaigne S, et al. Long-term human blood cultures: Application to circulating progenitor cell autografting. Bone Marrow Transplant 1987;2:67-72.

11. Freireich EJ, Levin RH, Whang J, et al. The function and fate of transfused leukocytes from donors with chronic myelocytic leukemia in leukopenic recipients. Ann NY Acad Sci 1964;113:1081-9.

12. Haines ME, Goldman JM, Worsley AM, et al. Chemotherapy and autografting for chronic granulocytic leukaemia in transformation: Probable prolongation of survival for some patients. Br J Haematol 1984;58:711-21.

13. Brito-Babapulle F, Apperly JF, Rassool F, et al. Complete remission after autografting for chronic myeloid leukaemia. Leuk Res 1987; 11:1115-17.

14. Storb R, Doney KC, Thomas ED. Marrow transplantation with or without donor buffy coat cells for 65 transfused aplastic anemia patients. Blood 1982;59:236-46.

15. Lasky LC, Ash RC, Kersey JH, et al. Collection of pluripotential hematopoietic stem cells by cytapheresis. Blood 1982;59:822-7.

16. Nguyen BT, Perkins HA. Quantitation of granulocyte-macrophage progenitor cells (CFU-C) in plateletpheresis and leukapheresis concentrates. Rev Fr Transfus Immunohematol 1979;22:489-500.

17. Lasky LC, Smith JA, McCullough J, Zanjani ED. Three-hour collection of committed and multipotent hematopoietic progenitor cells by apheresis. Transfusion 1987;27:276-8.

18. Körbling M, Dorken B, Ho AD, et al. Autologous transplantation of blood-derived hemopoietic stem cells after myeloablative therapy in a patient with Burkitt's lymphoma. Blood 1986;67:529-32.

19. Juttner CA, To LB, Ho JQ, et al. Early lympho-hemopoietic recovery after autografting using peripheral blood stem cells in acute non-lymphoblastic leukemia. Transplant Proc 1988;20:40-2.

20. Kessinger A, Armitage JO, Landmark JD, et al. Autologous peripheral hematopoietic stem cell transplantation restores hematopoietic function following marrow ablative therapy. Blood 1988;71:723-7.

21. Stiff PJ, Koester AR, Eagleton LE, et al. Autologous stem cell transplantation using peripheral blood stem cells. Transplantation 1987; 44:585-8.

22. Tilly H, Bastit D, Lucet JC, et al. Haemopoietic reconstitution after autologous peripheral blood stem cell transplantation in acute leukaemia (letter). Lancet 1986;2:154-5.

23. Law P, Dooley DC, Alsop P, et al. Density gradient isolation of peripheral blood mononuclear cells using a blood cell processor. Transfusion 1988;28:145-50.

24. Lasky LC, Hurd DD, Smith JA, Haake R. Peripheral blood stem cell collection and use in Hodgkin's disease. Comparison with marrow in autologous transplantation. Transfusion 1989;29:323-7.

25. Bostrom B, Moss TJ, Dehner LP, et al. Autologous peripheral blood stem cell transplantation in solid tumors. In: Dicke KA, Spitzer G, Jagannath S, Evinger-Hodges MJ, eds. Autologous bone marrow transplantation. Proceedings of the Fourth International Symposium. Houston: University of Texas, M.D. Anderson Cancer Center, 1989:707-11.

26. To LB, Russell J, Moore S, Juttner CA. Residual leukemia cannot be detected in very early remission peripheral blood stem cell collections in acute non-lymphoblastic leukemia. Leuk Res 1987;11:327-9.

27. Gorin NC. Collection, manipulation and freezing of haemopoietic stem cells. Clin Haematol 1986;15:19-48.

28. Stiff PJ, Murgo AJ, Zaroulis CG, et al. Unfractionated human marrow cell cryopreservation using dimethylsulfoxide and hydroxyethyl starch. Cryobiology 1983;20:17-24

29. Stiff PJ, Koester AR, Weidner MK, et al. Autologous bone marrow transplantation using unfractionated cells cryopreserved in dimethylsulfoxide and hydroxyethyl starch without controlled-rate freezing. Blood 1987;70:974.

30. To LB, Dyson PG, Branford AL, et al. Peripheral blood stem cells collected in very early remission produce rapid and sustained autologous haemopoietic reconstitution in acute non-lymphoblastic leukaemia. Bone Marrow Transplant 1987;2:103-8.

31. Spitzer G, Verma DS, Fisher R, et al. The myeloid progenitor cell--its value in predicting hematopoietic recovery after autologous bone marrow transplantation. Blood 1980;55:317-23.

32. To LB, Dyson PG, Branford AL, et al. CFU-MIX are no better than CFU-GM in predicting hemopoietic reconstitutive capacity of peripheral blood stem cells collected in the very early remission phase of acute nonlymphoblastic leukemia. Exp Hematol 1987;15:351-4.

33. To LB, Dyson PG, Juttner CA. Cell-dose effect in circulating stem-cell autografting (letter). Lancet 1986;2:404-5.

34. Reiffers J, Leverger G, Castaigne S, et al. Autologous blood stem cell transplantation in patients with haematological malignancies. Bone Marrow Transplant 1988;3(Supp. 1):167-8.

35. Lasky LC, Bostrom B, Smith J, et al. Clinical collection and use of peripheral blood stem cells in pediatric patients. Transplantation 1989;47:613-16.

36. Körbling M, Baumann M, Holdermann E, et al. Autologous blood stem cell transplantation (ABSCT) in 34 patients: its methodological advantage and limitation. Bone Marrow Transplant 1988;3(Supp 1): 51-3.

37. Leary AG, Ogawa M. Blast cell colony assay for umbilical cord blood and adult bone marrow progenitors. Blood 1987;69:953-6.

38. Heal JM, Brightman A. Exercise and circulating hematopoietic progenitor cells (CFU-GM) in humans. Transfusion 1987;27:115-18.

39. Lasky LC, Ascensao J, McCullough J, Zanjani ED. Steroid modulation of naturally occurring diurnal variation in circulating pluripotential haematopoietic cells (CFU-GEMM). Br J Haematol 1983;55:615-22.
40. Abboud CN, Brennan JK, Lichtman MA, Nusbacher J. Quantification of erythroid and granulocytic precursor cells in plateletpheresis residues. Transfusion 1980;20:9-16.
41. Cline MJ, Golde DW. Mobilization of hematopoietic stem cells (CFU-C) into the peripheral blood of man by endotoxin. Exp Hematol 1977;5:186-90.
42. Morra L, Ponassi A, Caristo G, et al. Comparison between diurnal changes and changes induced by hydrocortisone and epinephrine in circulating myeloid progenitor cells (CFU-GM) in man. Biomed Pharmacother 1984;38:167-70.
43. Ganser A, Bergmann M, Völkers B, et al. In vitro and in vivo effects of recombinant human erythropoietin on human hemopoietic progenitor cells. Contrib Nephrol 1988;66:123-30.
44. Socinski MA, Elias A, Schnipper L, et al. Granulocyte-macrophage colony stimulating factor expands the circulating haemopoietic progenitor cell compartment in man. Lancet 1988;1:1194-8.
45. Stiff PJ, Murgo AJ, Wittes RE, et al. Quantification of the peripheral blood colony forming unit-culture rise following chemotherapy: Could leukocytaphereses replace bone marrow for autologous transplantation? Transfusion 1983;23:500-3.
46. Richman CM, Weiner RS, Yankee RA. Increase in circulating stem cells following chemotherapy in man. Blood 1976;47:1031-9.
47. Castaigne S, Calvo F, Douay L, et al. Successful haematopoietic reconstitution using autologous peripheral blood mononucleated cells in a patient with acute promyelocytic leukemia. Br J Haematol 1986;63:209-11.
48. Juttner CA, To LB, Haylock DN, et al. Circulating autologous stem cells collected in very early remission from acute non-lymphoblastic leukaemia produce prompt but incomplete haemopoietic reconstitution after high dose melphalan or supralethal chemoradiotherapy. Br J Haematol 1985;61:739-45.
49. Reiffers J, Marit G, David B, et al. Autologous blood stem cell transplantation in acute myeloid leukaemia. Lancet 1988;1:419.
50. Reiffers J, Bernard P, David B, et al. Successful autologous transplantation with peripheral blood hemopoietic cells in a patient with acute leukemia. Exp Hematol 1986;14:312-15.
51. Laporte JP, Gorin NC, Feuchtenbaum J, et al. Relapse after autografting with peripheral blood stem cells (letter). Lancet 1987;2:1393-4.
52. Bell AJ, Figes A, Oscier DG, Hamblin TJ. Peripheral blood stem cell autografting (letter). Lancet 1986;1:1027-8.
53. Author names not printed. Use of circulating stem cells to accelerate myeloid recovery after autologous bone marrow transplantation (letter). Br J Haematol 1987;62:252-3.

54. Bell AJ, Figes A, Oscier DG, Hamblin TJ. Peripheral blood stem cell autografts in the treatment of lymphoid malignancies: Initial experience in three patients. Br J Haematol 1987;66:63-8.
55. Körbling M, Martin H, Fliedner TM. Autologous blood stem cell transplantation. In: Gale RP, Champlin C, eds. Progress in bone marrow transplantation. New York: Alan R. Liss, 1987:877-88.
56. Lasky LC, Fox SB, Smith JA, Bostrom B. Collection and use of peripheral blood stem cells in very small pediatric patients. Bone Marrow Transplant 1991;7:281-4.
57. Poynton CH. T-cell depletion in bone marrow transplantation. Bone Marrow Transplant 1988;3:265-79.
58. Dooley DC, Law P, Alsop P. A new density gradient for the separation of large quantities of rosette-positive and rosette-negative cells. Exp Hematol 1987;15:296-303.
59. Kessinger A, Smith DM, Strandjord SE, et al. Allogeneic transplantation of blood-derived, T cell-depleted hemopoietic stem cells after myeloablative treatment in a patient with acute lymphoblastic leukemia. Bone Marrow Transplant 1989;4:643-6.
60. Peters WP, Kurtzberg J, Atwater S, et al. The use of recombinant human granulocyte-macrophage colony-stimulating factor in autologous bone marrow transplantation. Prog Clin Biol Res 1990; 338: 121-8.
61. Lopez M, Pouillart P, Du Puy Montbrun MC, et al. Fast hematological reconstitution after combined infusion of autologous bone marrow purged with mafosfamide and autologous peripheral blood stem cells in a patient with Ewing sarcoma (letter). Bone Marrow Transplant 1988;3:172-4.
62. Agah R, Malloy B, Kerner M, Mazumder A. Generation and characterization of IL-2-activated bone marrow cells as a potent graft vs tumor effector in transplantation. J Immunol 1989;143:3093-9.
63. Blaise D, Olive D, Stoppa AM, et al. Hematologic and immunologic effects of the systemic administration of recombinant interleukin-2 after autologous bone marrow transplantation. Blood 1990;76:1092-7.
64. Charak BS, Malloy B, Agah R, Mazumder A. A novel approach to purging of leukemia by activation of bone marrow with interleukin 2. Bone Marrow Transplant 1990;6:193-8.
65. Lasky LC. Hematopoietic reconstitution using progenitors recovered from blood. Transfusion 1989;29:552-7.

In: Sacher RA, Brubaker DB, Kasprisin DO and McCarthy LJ, eds.
Cellular and Humoral Immunotherapy and Apheresis
Arlington, VA: American Association of Blood Banks, 1991

7

Extracorporeal Photopheresis

Howard K. Koh, MD, FACP

E XTRACORPOREAL PHOTOPHERESIS IS AN innovative treatment modality introduced by Edelson and colleagues in 1987[1,2] that is now a treatment of choice for one form of cutaneous T-cell lymphoma (CTCL). It also holds promise for efficacy in other diseases characterized by expanded populations of neoplastic or autoreactive T lymphocytes. Although its precise mechanism of action is unclear, photopheresis appears to work as a form of immunomodulation and immunoenhancement. This chapter outlines the evolution and present state of the art of extracorporeal photopheresis in the treatment of CTCL, summarizes the animal and immunologic experiments exploring mechanisms for this treatment and comments on possible new indications and ongoing clinical trials of photopheresis in other immune-related diseases.

The Evolution of Extracorporeal Photopheresis in the Treatment of Cutaneous T-Cell Lymphoma

Recognition of the special biologic properties of psoralen when combined with ultraviolet A light (PUVA) created the clinical discipline of photochemotherapy, from which extracorporeal photopheresis has evolved. Psoralens are naturally occurring tricyclic compounds that are biologically inert.[2,3] However, exposure of psoralens to UVA (320-400 nm) light causes their transient photoexcitation to a triplet state whose half-life is in the microsecond range.

Subsequently, activated psoralens can intercalate with cellular DNA (nuclear, mitochondrial and cell membrane) and other targets to form

Howard K. Koh, MD, FACP, Associate Professor of Dermatology, Medicine and Public Health, Departments of Dermatology and Medicine and the Section of Epidemiology and Biostatistics, Boston University Schools of Medicine and Public Health, Boston, Massachusetts mono- and bifunctional adducts to pyrimidine bases, causing inhibition of DNA synthesis and cell damage.[2-4]

In the early 1970's, researchers first used PUVA for the treatment of psoriasis, a common benign skin disorder characterized clinically by cutaneous plaques with thick scale and pathophysiologically by proliferation of epidermal cells. In this protocol, psoriasis patients ingest 8-methoxypsoralen (8-MOP) and (when psoralen levels peak in the blood 2 hours later), receive UVA rays while standing in a light box. In 1974, Parrish and colleagues[5] showed that PUVA caused complete clearing of severe, otherwise resistant, generalized psoriasis in 21 patients, with no major side effects. Subsequent studies have documented particular PUVA effects on T lymphocytes.[6]

Cutaneous T-cell lymphoma is an uncommon non-Hodgkin's lymphoma of the skin, characterized by mature CD4+ malignant lymphoid cells. Early stage CTCL can be indolent but late-stage disease is often aggressive and fatal. The clinical similarities of CTCL to psoriasis and the documented susceptibility of T cells to PUVA led researchers to hypothesize that PUVA could also successfully treat CTCL. In the late 1970's, Gilchrest and colleagues[7,8] showed that PUVA caused remission rates of 90% or more in early CTCL, with less successful responses in late-stage disease (tumors or erythroderma). Other studies have since confirmed that PUVA is a well-tolerated palliative therapy for CTCL, though concomitant treatment may be required in many cases.

CTCL can progress through a number of stages, including a particularly aggressive, erythrodermic phase called Sézary syndrome.[9] In this syndrome, large numbers of clonally derived malignant CD4+ T cells [characterized by hyperconvoluted nuclei (Sézary cells)] circulate in both the blood and skin, causing a T-cell lymphoma-leukemia. Patients with the Sézary form of CTCL have widespread cutaneous erythroderma, associated cutaneous discomfort and pain, hand and foot keratoderma with fissuring and superinfection, and adenopathy. In addition to this extreme morbidity, Sézary syndrome carries a median survival of under 3 years.[9]

Until recently, there were few effective treatments for Sézary syndrome.[9] Edelson and others[10,11] first showed that leukapheresis could palliate patients with Sézary syndrome, since removing malignant T cells from vascular components promoted subsequent cell migration from soft tissues, leading to a decrease in erythroderma and pruritus. However, leukapheresis usually required frequent administration (two to four times per week). Edelson et al[1,2] then reasoned that since PUVA therapy was effective in CTCL, concentrating PUVA therapy directly on white cells of Sézary syndrome patients (extracorporeal photochemotherapy or photopheresis) and bypassing shielding effects of the skin might improve cell kill. Hence, they devised a protocol that combined leukapheresis and PUVA; this directed therapy theoretically would have no effect on nonnuclear blood components such as red cells, platelets and plasma proteins. In this protocol, patients ingested 8-MOP orally in the standard fashion

(0.6 mg/kg) and then 2 hours later their blood was removed through an intravenous cannula. Centrifuge techniques collected the buffy coat, which was then diluted in saline and the patient's own psoralen-rich plasma, irradiated through a UVA field outside the body and finally reinfused back into the patient. Edelson et al chose to expose blood to 1-2 J/cm^2 UVA in the presence of 100 ng/mL of 8-MOP, since this regimen almost completely blocked T-cell division. Measurements of monoclonal antibody to DNA psoralen photoadducts documented ongoing photomodification.[1] They arbitrarily chose a conservative treatment regimen of two consecutive days a month.

The results of this clinical study were published in 1987 by Edelson et al[1,2] who treated 37 patients with Sézary syndrome (28 men and 9 women). All of these patients had failed previous therapies. Patients with visceral disease were excluded. Seventy-three percent (27/37) showed improvement (>25%) in skin erythroderma. Of these, nine had more than 75% clearing and two patients maintained long-term complete remissions up to 29 months after all treatment had been discontinued. Erythroderma, hand and foot keratoderma, and skin itching and pain all improved, leading to a better quality of life. Eight of 10 patients with lymphomatous lymph node involvement and 19 of 27 with dermatopathic lymph nodes responded.

Laboratory results in this study showed that in 11 clinically improved patients with clonal disease (identified by abnormal karyotype or T-cell receptor beta-chain gene rearrangement), photopheresis did not eliminate this clone. Also, repeat skin biopsies in patients reaching complete remission showed microscopic persistence of atypical cells. However, in six clinically improved patients who initially had greater than 90% T4 cells, the overall T4/T8 ratio decreased with treatment. In five patients with high numbers of BE2+ markers (a late activation T-cell marker associated with CTCL), the proportions of these marked cells decreased (from a mean of 26% to 5%). In addition, the lymphocyte viability of extracorporeally irradiated lymphocytes (as judged by trypan blue exclusion) dropped from 91% to 12% after 72 hours' incubation ("slow kill"). In sum, these laboratory data substantiated reversal of the disease process, though cure could not be documented. Without a control group, it is difficult to determine the impact of photopheresis on survival; however, a recent update by Edelson[12] notes that the median survival of these 27 responding patients is now 43.5 months (with 2/3 still alive), greater than the anticipated 30 months in historical controls.

Most notably in this study, photopheresis was well-tolerated without the severe side effects traditionally seen with chemotherapy. Other than transient hypotension, there were no significant side effects. There were several episodes of herpetic infection but no other major opportunistic infection; delayed type hypersensitivity (as measured by skin testing) was normal and general immunocompetence appeared unaffected.

The degree of improvement seen in these otherwise refractory patients and other observations led Edelson et al[1,2] to postulate that immunologic mechanisms, and not simply cytoreductive mechanisms, explained the clinical results of photopheresis. These proposed immunologic mechanisms are discussed below.

Photopheresis is now available at over 40 centers in the United States and abroad. The UVAR system (produced by Therakos, Westchester, PA, a subsidiary of Johnson & Johnson) allows photopheresis therapy to be delivered at the bedside through a single portable apparatus that one can operate using an attached computerized panel.[13] In the UVAR system, blood is shunted into a 250-cc centrifuge bowl and over six cycles, 240 cc total of leukocyte-enriched buffy coat are collected and mixed with 300 mL of the patient's psoralen-rich plasma and 200 mL of sterile normal saline (see Fig 7-1). Then this mixture is irradiated for 270 minutes as it circulates through a 1.4-mm thick fluid path in a photoceptor cassette (a UVA transparent acrylic unit). As each patient's blood is shunted through his/her own disposable photoceptor apparatus, there is no cross contam-

THE PROCESS OF PHOTOPHERESIS

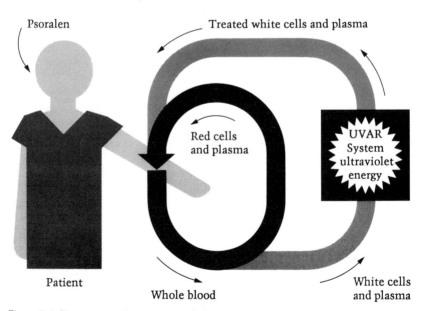

Figure 7-1. The process of extracorporeal photopheresis.

ination of blood and no possibility of transmission of AIDS or other blood-borne diseases.

Further Studies and Questions Regarding Photopheresis in Cutaneous T-Cell Lymphoma

Since Edelson's initial study, two other studies have confirmed the efficacy of photopheresis in CTCL. Heald[14] and colleagues reported that in 22 erythrodermic Sézary patients (19 of whom had no previous therapy), five cleared substantially (over 75% skin involvement) and another 10 had moderate clearing (25% to 75%). Major toxicity was limited to recurrent herpetic infection in one patient. Heald and colleagues note that when comparing the five best responders to the five worst responders, shorter duration of disease (<1 vs >1 year) and lower CD4/CD8 ratios (5.27 for responders vs 39.6 for nonresponders) correlated with clinical response. They speculate, therefore, that perhaps only immunocompetent patients with short duration of disease can respond to this presumably immuno-enhancing maneuver.

Armus et al[15] showed that photopheresis caused complete or partial response in seven of eight CTCL patients. While Edelson et al[1] and Heald et al[14] concentrated on treating erythrodermic CTCL patients, Armus et al[15] noted clinical response in all three nonerythrodermic patients treated (with tumor, extensive plaque or patch stage disease). We await more definitive data from other centers to document the clinical effects of photopheresis in all subsets of CTCL.

In sum, these studies show that perhaps up to 75% of patients with Sézary syndrome respond to photopheresis. However, only a quarter or so achieve complete remission (100% disappearance of disease lasting for at least 1 month) on photopheresis alone. For these responding patients, the erythroderma usually improves slowly (over a 5- to 6-month period). In addition, for those patients who reach only partial remission on pho-topheresis alone, it is as yet unclear whether the addition of a second agent, (such as low-dose oral methotrexate, interferon, topical nitrogen mustard or azothiaprine), can improve response. Clearly, one hopes to boost, and not block, the presumed immunoenhancement of photophere-sis by adding such therapies. More data are needed.

It should also be noted that until recently, photopheresis has utilized crystalline 8-MOP, which is erratically absorbed. Recently, the use of a gelatin capsule formulation (Oxsoralen Ultra®) has become preferred over the crystalline formulation because of its more reliable and rapid absorp-tion.[16] Also, measuring 8-MOP levels in the treatment bag is thought to reflect the levels more accurately over several apheresis cycles, as com-pared to a serum level at a single point in time.[16] As other forms of psoralen are more water soluble and have higher DNA binding affinity, they may ultimately improve the efficacy of photopheresis.[3]

Investigations Into the Mechanisms of Extracorporeal Photopheresis

Several observations suggest that photopheresis works through immunomodulation. Photopheresis treats only 10%-15% of all white cells,[13] yet this limited nonspecific insult results in a clinically significant, apparently clone-specific, suppression without affecting other T cells and causing general immunoincompetence. A recent update notes that some patients with Sézary syndrome treated with photopheresis have maintained complete remission up to 7 years after discontinuation of treatment.[12] Also, since intense leukapheresis does not cause the degree of clinical improvement seen with photopheresis, the return of photodamaged cells appears to be the critical step.[17]

This has led Edelson and others to speculate that photopheresis acts as a form of "T-cell vaccination," whereby the reintroduction of an attenuated, damaged pathogen induces clonotypic suppression presumably via cells that bear anti-idiotypic receptors to the T-cell clone.[11,18]

Interventions in animal studies by Cohen[19] and colleagues show parallels to photopheresis. Their studies demonstrate a capacity to ameliorate or prevent autoimmune disease by the in vitro administration of lethally damaged, syngeneic, pathogenic T-cell clones. The experimental autoimmune encephalomyelitis (EAE) model, a rat model similar to multiple sclerosis (MS) in humans has received the most attention. EAE, leading to paralysis and death associated with a T-cell infiltration of the central nervous system, can be invoked in rats by injecting myelin basic protein (MBP) antigen in complete Freund's adjuvant. Anti-MBP clones can be isolated from sacrificed rats. Subsequent injection of those T-cell clones in naive rats can also lead to EAE and paralysis. However, if after isolation, those pathogenic T-cell clones are first damaged (by pressure, glutaraldehyde or other means) and then injected into naive rats, subsequent challenge by introduction of MBP antigen protects the rats from paralysis or EAE and the animals remain healthy.

Khavari et al[20] have since shown extracorporeal PUVA to be more effective than glutaraldehyde or pressure in causing this vaccination effect in EAE rats. In exploring the pathophysiology, Gasparro et al[3] have shown that the doses of 8-MOP (100 ng/mL) and UVA (1 J/cm^2) used in photopheresis cripple T-cell proliferative processes (as measured by tritiated thymidine incorporation) while leaving cell membrane integrity (as measured by trypan blue exclusion) modified but initially intact. Hence, photopheresis presents intact but inactivated cells to the immune system over a several-day period.[21] It is hypothesized that the T-cell damage at this level may be gentle enough to enhance expression of clonotypic antigens but severe enough to stimulate clearing by an unaffected reticuloendothelial system. The most obvious candidate for photomodification is the T-cell receptor(TCR), which is uniquely antigenic for each T-cell clone and whose purpose is to bind to appropriately presented foreign antigens. Either direct photo-modification or changes affecting processing or presentation to TCRs may be involved.

More direct work with photopheresis in animal studies support an immunologic mechanism. Berger[22,23] and colleagues have evaluated the effects of reinfusion of phototreated autoimmune lymphocytes in the MRL/1 mouse model of systemic lupus erythematosus. Such mice homozygous for the 1pr mutation exhibit early onset of autoimmune disease with massive lymphadenopathy and splenomegaly caused by proliferation of phenotypically abnormal, benign inducer T cells. Berger et al[23] evaluated the introduction of phototreated syngeneic splenocytes (incubated with 100 ng/mL of 8-MOP and 1 J/cm^2 of UVA) into young recipient MRL/1 mice as a prophylactic measure and into older mice with active disease as a therapeutic measure. They evaluated these effects by monitoring in vitro endpoints (anti-DNA antibody production and T-cell hyperproliferation and mitogen assays) and in vivo endpoints (lymphoid organomegaly and survival). Infusion of photoinactivated lymphocytes showed improvements of all the above-mentioned endpoints in younger mice treated prophylactically. However, while some parameters improved in older mice with active disease (reduced lymphoid hyperplasia and decreased double-stranded DNA antibody production) other parameters did not (no improvement in renal disease and survival). Taken together, these and other studies by Berger et al[22] demonstrated that infusion of phototreated autoimmune lymphocytes caused suppression of immunoactive cells while preserving generalized immunocompetence. The effect depended on the presence of intact cells or membranes (since lysed phototreated cells were not effective) and the presence of a relatively intact immune system.

Perez et al[24,25] demonstrated the effects of photopheresis-like intervention in skin transplantation in mice. In this study, they grafted CBA/j mouse donor skin transplants onto BALB/c mice to introduce histoincompatible tissue with disparity in the H-2 locus. After graft rejection, spleens from recipient mice were removed and processed into single-cell suspensions. These splenocytes were then incubated with 100 ng/mL of 8-MOP and exposed to 1 J/cm^2 UVA to generate photoinactivated effector T cells or "PET" cells. After the PET cells were subsequently infused into naive BALB/c mice, the recipient mice were tested for specific T-cell immunoresponsiveness to CBA/j alloantigens (compared to control irrelevant alloantigens) according to in vitro endpoints [mixed lymphocyte culture (MLC), cytotoxicity (CTL)] and in vivo endpoints [delayed type hypersensitivity (DTH) and challenge with fresh CBA/j skin allograft]. Their results showed that compared to controls treated BALB/c recipients had: 1) poorer MLC proliferation, 2) lower CTL responses to CBA/j alloantigens, 3) suppressed DTH responses and, most importantly, 4) longer retention of CBA/j skin grafts. Hence, they could induce hyporeactivity against a specific set of major histocompatibility complex antigens by photoinactivating and introducing syngeneic effector cells.[24,25] Further experiments suggested that the induction of an antigen-specific inhibitory cell population, and not deletion of effector T-cell populations, was responsible for inducing this hyporeactivity. Ongoing research is seeking to identify further this inhibitory cell population.

The Use of Photopheresis in Other Immune-Related Diseases

There is now growing interest that photopheresis may be effective in other immune-related diseases marked by clonal expansion of aberrant T cells.

A recently completed Phase III multicenter trial has demonstrated the efficacy of photopheresis in progressive systemic sclerosis (PSS). This disorder is marked by thickening and hardening of the skin (with infiltration of involved tissue by activated T lymphocytes) sometimes associated with dysfunction of the esophagus, lungs and kidneys. A pilot study of photopheresis treating two patients with rapidly progressive PSS showed that this treatment reduced the cutaneous thickening.[26]

This finding prompted a randomized control trial[27] in which 80 patients with steadily advancing PSS (progression of cutaneous thickening by ≥30% in the previous year with total disease duration <4 years) were randomized to either photopheresis or D-penicillamine (up to 750 mg/day) for 6 months. Blinded observers evaluated skin thickness and surface area scores, Raynaud's phenomenon, collagen thickness on serial skin biopsies, pulmonary function tests and other parameters. Preliminary results on 43 evaluable patients showed 77% (17/22) of those treated with photopheresis improved their skin severity score (compared to baseline) as opposed to 33% (7/21) of patients treated with D-penicillamine. The mean skin severity score for patients on photopheresis improved over baseline, whereas the score for those in the D-penicillamine group did not. Serial skin biopsies showed a decrease in dermal collagen, but pulmonary function tests were largely unchanged. Most important, the side effects necessitating cessation of treatment occurred in only 1/35 patients in the photopheresis arm versus 6/29 in the D-penicillamine arm. We are awaiting FDA approval for photopheresis as a treatment of progressive systemic sclerosis.

Rook et al[28] recently published a short report on the efficacy of photopheresis in four patients with pemphigus vulgaris, an autoimmune blistering disease of the skin and mucous membranes characterized by IgG antibody against a 130 kD epidermal protein. Photopheresis led to clinical improvement in two of four patients, with a reduction in their concurrent cytotoxic (high dose cytoxan and prednisone) therapy. The clinical response was paralleled by decreases in the serum antiepidermal cell antibody.

Bisaccia et al[29] published preliminary results in a single-arm pilot study of photopheresis in AIDS-related complex. This study treated 5 HIV+ patients and showed disappearance of adenopathy (5), increases in p24 and gp120 antibodies (5), resolution of symptoms (4) and negative HIV cultures (2). We await confirmation of these results in a larger study.

Vonderheid et al[30] noted some efficacy of photopheresis in four patients with refractory psoriasis, two of whom had concomitant methotrexate treatment. Peripheral blood lymphocytes in these treated patients lost capacity to produce interleukin-2 in vitro. However, a recent report by Wilfert et al[31] showed minimal effects of photopheresis in psoriatic arthritis.

Photopheresis has minimal clinical effects in preliminary studies of B-cell chronic lymphocytic leukemia.[32]

Ongoing photopheresis trials include patients with rheumatoid arthritis (an autoimmune disease where oligoclonal expansion of T lymphocytes may play a role),[33] cardiac transplantation, multiple sclerosis and HTLV-I+ adult T-cell leukemia (see Table 7-1).

Summary and Future Directions

Photopheresis is a new, nontoxic form of therapy that appears to cause specific T-cell regulation. Presently, it is an effective form of treatment for erythrodermic CTCL/Sézary syndrome and will likely become a treatment option for progressive systemic sclerosis.

However, as the field of photopheresis is in its infancy, many clinical and laboratory questions remain unanswered. We need more information about optimal dose-response schedules to maximize clinical response. We must learn which clinical and laboratory variables best predict response to photopheresis treatment. We need more information about response duration and how to extend it. We do not yet know how to combine photopheresis with other therapies. Refinements in the type and delivery of psoralen might make treatment more efficient. Ideally, we need to

Table 7-1. Current Photopheresis Protocols

1. HTLV-I + acute T-cell leukemia/lymphoma
2. Cardiac transplantation
3. Rheumatoid arthritis
4. Multiple sclerosis
5. Pemphigus vulgaris
6. Progressive systemic sclerosis
7. Systemic lupus erythematosus
8. Graft-vs-host disease
9. Type 1 diabetes mellitus

improve this modality to induce even more selective targeted killing. Hopefully, further research can reveal the precise mechanisms of photopheresis to maximize its future use in human disease.

References

1. Edelson RL, Berger C, Gasparro F, et al. Treatment of cutaneous T-cell lymphoma by extracorporeal photochemotherapy. N Engl J Med 1987;316:297-303.
2. Edelson R. Light activated drugs. Sci Am 1988;259:68-75.
3. Gasparro FP, Dall'Amico R, Goldminz D, et al. Molecular aspects of extracorporeal photochemotherapy. Yale J Biol Med 1989;62:579-93.
4. Gasparro F, Dall'Amico R, O'Malley M, et al. Cell membrane DNA: A new target for psoralen photoadduct formation. Photochem Photobiol 1990;52:315-21.
5. Parrish JA, Fitzpatrick TB, Tannenbaum L, et al. Photochemotherapy of psoriasis with oral methoxsalen and long wavelength ultraviolet light. N Engl J Med 1974;29:1207-11.
6. Morison W, Parrish JA, McAuliffe DJ, Bloch RJ. Sensitivity of mononuclear cells to PUVA: Effect on subsequent stimulation with antigens and on exclusion of trypan blue dyes. Clin Exp Dermatol 1981; 6:273-7.
7. Gilchrest BA, Parrish JA, Tanenbaum L, et al. Oral methoxsalen photochemotherapy of mycosis fungoides. Cancer 1976;38:683-89.
8. Gilchrest BA. Methoxsalen photochemotherapy for mycosis fungoides. Cancer Treat Rep 1979;63:663-67.
9. Wieselthier JS, Koh HK. Sézary syndrome: Diagnosis, prognosis, and critical review of treatment options. J Am Acad Dermatol 1990; 22:381-401.
10. Edelson R, Facktor M, Andrews A, et al. Successful management of the Sézary syndrome: Mobilization and removal of extravascular neoplastic T cells by leukopheresis. N Engl J Med 1974;291:293-4.
11. Pineda A, Winkelmann R. Leukapheresis in the treatment of Sézary syndrome. J Am Acad Dermatol 1981;5:544-9.
12. Edelson RL. Photopheresis: A new therapeutic concept. Yale J Biol Med 1989;62:565-77.
13. Lee KH, Garro J. Engineering aspects of extracorporeal photochemotherapy. Yale J Biol Med 1989;62:621-28.
14. Heald PW, Perez MI, Christensen I, et al. Photopheresis therapy of cutaneous T-cell lymphoma: The Yale-New Haven Hospital experience. Yale J Biol Med 1989;62:629-38.
15. Armus S, Keyes B, Cahill C, et al. Photopheresis for the treatment of cutaneous T cell lymphoma. J Am Acad Dermatol 1990;23:898-902.
16. Heald PW, Perez MI, Gasparro FP. Dosage guidelines: Extracorporeal photochemotherapy (photopheresis). Arch Dermatol 1990;126:1369.

17. Edelson RL. Photopheresis. J Clin Apheresis 1990;5:77-9.
18. Miyasaka N. T-cell vaccination. Clin Immunol 1989;21:1121-7.
19. Cohen IR. Regulation of autoimmune disease: Physiological and therapeutic. Immunol Rev 1986;94:5.
20. Khavari PA, Edelson RL, Lider O, et al. Specific vaccination against photoinactivated cloned T cells. Clin Res 1988;36:662.
21. Heald P, Perez M, McKieran G, et al. Extracorporeal photochemotherapy: Indications, methodology, safety aspects, side effects and long-term results. J Photodermatol 1989;6:171-6.
22. Berger C. Experimental murine and primate models for dissection of the immunosuppressive potential of photochemotherapy in autoimmune disease and transplantation. Yale J Biol Med 1989;62:611-20.
23. Berger CL, Perez M, Laroche L, Edelson R. Inhibition of autoimmune disease in a murine model of systemic lupus erythematosus induced by exposure to syngeneic photoinactivated lymphocytes. J Invest Dermatol 1990;94:52-7.
24. Perez M, Edelson R, Laroche L, Berger C. Inhibition of antiskin allograft immunity by infusions with syngeneic photoinactivated effector lymphocytes. J Invest Dermatol 1989;92:669-76.
25. Perez M, Edelson RL, John L, et al. Inhibition of antiskin allograft immunity induced by infusion with photoinactivated and effector T lymphocytes (PET cells). Yale J Biol Med 1989;62:575-610.
26. Rook A, Freundlich B, Nahass GT, et al. Treatment of autoimmune disease with extracorporeal photochemotherapy: Progressive systemic sclerosis—preliminary report. Yale J Biol Med 1989;62:639-46.
27. Rook AH, Freundlich B, Edelson R, et al. Effective treatment of progressive systemic sclerosis (PSS) with extracorporeal photochemotherapy. Clin Res 1990;38:420.
28. Rook AH, Jegasothy BV, Heald P, et al. Extracorporeal photochemotherapy for drug-resistant pemphigus vulgaris. Ann Intern Med 1990;112:303-5.
29. Bisaccia E, Berger C, Klainer AS. Extracorporeal photopheresis in the treatment of AIDS-related complex: A pilot study. Ann Intern Med 1990;113:270-5.
30. Vonderheid EC, Kang C, Kadin M, et al. Extracorporeal photopheresis in psoriasis vulgaris: Clinical and immunologic observations. J Am Acad Dermatol 1990;3:703-12.
31. Wilfert H, Honigsmann H, Steiner G, et al. Treatment of psoriatic arthritis by extracorporeal photochemotherapy. Br J Dermatol 1990; 122:225-32.
32. Knobler RM, Pirker R, Kokoschka EM, et al. Experimental treatment of chronic lymphocytic leukemia with extracorporeal photochemotherapy. Blut 1990;60:215-18.
33. Stamenkovic I, Stegagno M, Wright KA, et al. Clonal dominance among T-lymphocyte infiltrates in arthritis. Proc Natl Acad Sci USA 1988;85:1179-83.

In: Sacher RA, Brubaker DB, Kasprisin DO and McCarthy LJ, eds.
Cellular and Humoral Immunotherapy and Apheresis
Arlington, VA: American Association of Blood Banks, 1991

8

The Future of Cellular Immunotherapy of Cancer

Alexander Fefer, MD; John A. Thompson, MD;
Carl M. Higuchi, MD; and Catherine G. Lindgren

BOUT 20 YEARS AGO, a number of animal models were developed in which cellular immunotherapy in the form of lymphocytes immune to tumor-associated antigens cured disseminated malignancy. The potential clinical relevance of those models was considered questionable partly because no targets on human tumors for immunologic attacks were known and partly because no one could imagine how the huge number of effector lymphocytes required for therapy could possibly be obtained. During the past 10 years there has been a marked resurgence of interest in cellular immunotherapy of cancer stimulated largely by: 1) advances in cellular and molecular immunology with a resultant increase in knowledge about murine and human T-cell subsets, about how antigens are processed and recognized and about the effector mechanisms mediating tumor eradication; 2) advances in DNA technology with the identification of a number of lymphokines, most notably IL-2, and their availability in large quantity for use in vitro and in vivo; 3) advances in tissue culture technology, which have made it possible to expand various types of lymphocytes and clone antigen-specific T cells, including some that could react to tumor-specific antigens in humans; 4) advances in the development of automated blood cell separators, which make it possible to obtain cells in large number for clinical trials; and 5) advances in

Alexander Fefer, MD, Professor of Medicine, University of Washington, Seattle, and Member, Fred Hutchinson Cancer Research Center, Seattle; John A. Thompson, MD, Assistant Professor of Medicine, University of Washington, Seattle; Carl M. Higuchi, MD, Assistant Professor of Medicine, University of Hawaii Cancer Center, Honolulu, Hawaii; and Catherine G. Lindgren, Staff Scientist, University of Washington, Seattle, Washington
(This research was supported by the National Institutes of Health grants CA 18029-16, 5 P01 CA47748-02, N01-CM-47668-02 and 2 T32 CA09515-6.)

clinical research with encouraging preliminary results using cellular immunotherapy in the form of lymphokine-activated killer (LAK) cells and tumor-infiltrating lymphocytes (TILs).

This chapter will review briefly some of the principles of cellular immunotherapy derived from murine models, comment on the preliminary results of cellular immunotherapy trials in humans and provide examples of the potential use of cellular immunotherapy in three different kinds of ongoing clinical trials at our institution. Some of the issues that must be resolved in order to devise cellular immunotherapy approaches that might be more effective and be more widely applicable to more cancer patients will thus be identified.

Animal Models for Cellular Immunotherapy Using Tumor-Specific T Cells

A number of animal models have been developed in which disseminated antigenic tumors can be eradicated by the adoptive transfer of T cells specifically immune to the tumor-associated antigens—especially as an adjunct to noncurative chemotherapy.[1-4] These models have served as a prototype of what might be achieved if the host immune response to an autologous tumor could be identified, selectively amplified and used in humans.

The most extensively studied model has involved the treatment of disseminated FBl-3, a Friend retrovirus-induced erythroleukemia, in C57BL/6 mice.[5] Mice inoculated intraperitoneally with FBL-3 on day 0 were treated on day 5, at a time when the leukemia cells are disseminated and detectable in the peripheral blood and lymphoid organs. Cumulative results of the original series of experiments, reported in 1972, are presented in Fig 8-1. Untreated mice died within 2 weeks, as did mice treated only with immune lymphocytes. Treatment with cyclophosphamide (CY, 180 mg/kg) alone, or with CY plus normal non-immune lymphocytes, or with CY plus lymphocytes immune to unrelated antigens prolonged survival to about 3 weeks but cured no mice. By contrast, treatment with CY plus cells immune to FBL-3 (ie, lymphocytes from syngeneic donors immunized to FBL-3) cured the vast majority of leukemic mice.

Subsequent studies [4,6-8] in this model as well as in other similar models yielded a series of observations related to successful immunotherapy: 1) donor T cells were required for therapeutic efficacy; 2) the T cells had to be immunologically specifically reactive to tumor-associated antigens and the encoded major histocompatibility complex (MHC) antigens; 3) the infused lymphocytes had to be able to proliferate and persist in the recipient for a long period of time; 4) therapeutic efficacy depended directly on the number of donor T cells infused, ie, the larger the number the greater the effect; 5) the T-cell growth factor interleukin-2 (IL-2) enhanced the growth of tumor-specific T cells in vitro and IL-2 in vivo

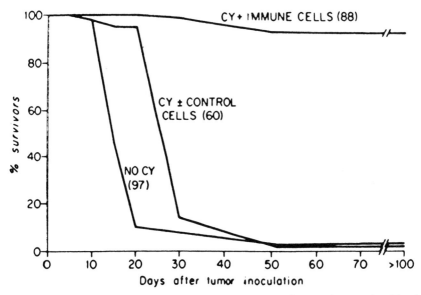

Figure 8-1. Summary of results of syngeneic adoptive chemoimmunotherapy of a Friend lymphoma (numbers in parentheses = number of tumor-bearing mice treated).

augmented the therapeutic efficacy of such adoptively transferred lymphocytes; 6) the generation of such cells in vitro and their therapeutic efficacy in vivo was further enhanced by restimulation in vitro with appropriate tumor antigen; and 7) both CD8[+] and CD4[+] T-cell subsets could mediate the immunologic eradication of tumor. The effector mechanism, however, was different for each subset. For example, the main mechanism by which CD4[+] T cells can eradicate tumor is by secreting lymphokines, which promotes the activity of other tumoricidal effector cells such as macrophages. By contrast, CD8[+] T cells recognize the tumor antigens in the context of Class 1 MHC molecules and lyse tumors directly with Class 1 restricted specificity.

Animal Models for Cellular Immunotherapy Using LAK Cells

The other effector cell that has received much attention for cellular immunotherapy studies in animals is a cell with LAK activity.[9] Murine lymphocytes cultured in pharmacologic concentrations of IL-2 for several days acquired the ability to lyse promiscuously a wide variety of tumor targets in a non-MHC restricted fashion with relative sparing of normal tissue. Such LAK activity is mediated by a heterogeneous population of cells rather than a single type of cell. Most LAK cells represent activated natural killer (NK) cells, but some may arise from T cells. For purposes of this chapter, we shall refer to LAK precursor (LAKp) cells, which, when cultured in IL-2, acquire LAK activity, or to LAK effector (LAKe) cells, which have direct LAK activity without requiring additional exposure to IL-2 in vitro.[9]

Extensive studies have demonstrated that LAK cells cause regression of established tumors and inhibit growth of pulmonary and hepatic metastases in syngeneic mice. In a series of studies in tumor-bearing mice,[10-13] LAK cells alone (without IL-2) had little therapeutic effect, whereas IL-2 alone had a significant therapeutic effect, especially if high doses of IL-2 were used. The infusion of a combination of exogenously generated LAK cells plus IL-2 was therapeutically most effective. A higher dose of IL-2 induced a greater LAK activity and antitumor effect in vivo. A larger number of LAK cells also exerted a greater antitumor effect. The efficacy of IL-2 ± LAK is, however, decreased by immunosuppressive agents such as corticosteroids, cyclosporin or radiation. The mechanism by which the therapeutic effect of IL-2 alone or IL-2 plus LAK cells is mediated, has not yet been definitively identified and may differ in different tumor models, perhaps depending on the degree of tumor immunogenicity. The effects might be mediated by LAK cells induced by IL-2 and/or by tumor-specific T lymphocytes augmented in number and activity by IL-2 and/or by secretion of other lympho-kines or cytokines in response to IL-2 ± lymphocytes. The mechanism by which LAK cells recognize, bind and selectively lyse malignant targets has yet to be identified. It is certainly possible that some heterogeneous tumors may contain some tumor cells that have become deficient in Class 1 molecules. Such tumor cells might no longer be susceptible to lysis by CD8+ T cells but might be susceptible to eradication by non-MHC-restricted LAK cells.

Cellular Immunotherapy Using LAK Cells in Humans

Cells with LAK activity have been generated from peripheral blood lymphocytes of normal people and cancer patients. Although some normal cells are also lysed,[14,15] LAK cells preferentially lyse malignant cells. LAK activity is operationally defined as the in vitro lysis of fresh autologous or allogeneic tumor cells or NK-resistant cultured tumor lines, such as Daudi. Most LAKe have the phenotypic characteristics of activated NK cells (CD56+, CD16+, CD3-), but some "NK-like" T cells that coexpress CD3 and NK markers can also mediate LAK activity.[16] Thus, LAK activity appears to be mediated by phenotypically heterogeneous and functionally diverse subpopulations of lymphocytes.[17] Among the targets that have been shown to be susceptible to lysis by LAK cells are fresh tumor cells obtained from patients with acute myeloid leukemia, acute lymphoblastic leukemia, chronic myelogenous leukemia (CML) or malignant lymphoma.[18-21] Such susceptibility is non-cell-cycle specific and is maintained in cell lines that demonstrate pleiotropic drug resistance markers.[22,23] In addition to being directly lytic, LAK cells also inhibit malignant colony proliferation in assays of clonogenic tumor growth.[24,25] LAK cells have little or no effect on hematologic progenitors in vitro.

In Phase I/II clinical trials with a variety of IL-2 preparations and regimens ± LAK cells, objective tumor responses have been reported in some patients with advanced malignancies, especially metastatic renal cell carcinoma and melanoma.[26-29] In the largest reported trial of IL-2 plus exogenously generated autologous LAK cells[30] various patients with metastatic malignancies unresponsive to conventional therapy or for which no conventional effective therapy is available were treated with a very high dose of IL-2 given by bolus injection every 8 hours on days 1-5. After a 2-day recovery period, the patients underwent leukapheresis daily on days 8-12. The lymphocytes collected were cultured in IL-2 for 3-4 days and were then reinfused into the patients on days 13-15; the same IL-2 regimen was administered on days 13-17. This approach has now been used by the National Cancer Institute to treat several hundred cancer patients. Approximately 20% of melanoma patients have exhibited at least a partial response (PR), defined as at least 50% tumor shrinkage, and approximately 30% of renal cell carcinoma patients have responded, including about 8% who had a complete response (CR), ie, complete disappearance of all evidence of tumor.

These results, though very encouraging, have not yet been fully reproduced by others. Thus, a six-center study using the same Rosenberg IL-2/LAK regimen to treat patients with renal cell carcinoma failed to yield a comparably high response rate (only 16% of patients responded).[31] A trial performed collaboratively by 14 institutions with the same Rosenberg IL-2/LAK regimen had only about a 12% response rate.[32] The reason for the differences is not yet known, but is assumed to reflect some differences in patient selection.

IL-2 administered in high doses is toxic. The frequent toxicities include fever, nausea, vomiting and diarrhea, skin rash, mild hepatic dysfunction, thrombocytopenia and a capillary leak syndrome characterized by hypotension, fluid retention, oliguria with azotemia and respiratory distress. Less common toxicities include bacterial infections, neurologic complications such as confusion and seizures, arrhythmias and cardiac ischemia.[30,33,34] The toxicity of therapy with IL-2 plus LAK cells is attributable almost totally to the IL-2.[28,30,35]

The treatment regimens that have induced the highest response rates have tended to be the most toxic ones. However, the relationship between IL-2 dose with or without LAK cells and the immunomodulatory and antitumor effects in patients is not clear because of the heterogeneity of the patients treated and of the IL-2 regimens used.[27,30,33,35-37]

We have conducted three sequential trials of IL-2 (Roche) plus LAK cells in an effort to decrease the toxicity of the therapy, determine the relationship between IL-2 dose and therapeutic efficacy, study ways to maximize the number of LAK cells generated for infusion and determine whether a low-dose maintenance phase of IL-2 would be tolerable and beneficial. The IL-2 was administered by continuous intravenous infusion instead of by bolus injection because of the demonstration that IL-2 induces greater immunomodulatory effects when administered by CIV infusion than when administered by bolus injection.[33]

In the first trial[28] IL-2 was administered at 3×10^6 U/m^2/day on days 1-5 (induction) and days 13-17 (maintenance). Leukapheresis was performed on days 8-10 with reinfusion of LAK cells on days 13-15. Of eight patients evaluable for tumor response, one responded with a CR, which endures at 38+ months.

In the second trial[28] the dose of IL-2 was doubled. Patients received IL-2 at 6×10^6 U/m^2/day on days 1-5 and 12-16, underwent leukapheresis on days 7-9 and received LAK cells on days 12-14. In an effort to increase the number of LAK cells generated, the first leukapheresis was performed one day earlier, at a time of peak rebound peripheral lymphocytosis, thus eliminating the Ficoll-Hypaque purification of lymphocytes. An average of 1.9×10^{11} LAK cells were infused per patient (27.5×10^5 lytic units/patient). Five of 20 patients responded (three CR for 33+, 25+ and 14+ months, and two PR for 31+ and 9 months). The dose limiting toxicity was most severe during maintenance, so that >70% of patients required Intensive Care Unit support, and 100% of the planned maintenance dose could not be given.

Since a longer maintenance phase of IL-2 given in conjunction with LAK cells might be beneficial and since less IL-2 might be required to maintain than to induce LAK activity in vivo, a third trial[38] was initiated in which patients received IL-2 at 6×10^6 U/m^2/day on days 1-5, underwent leukapheresis on days 7-9 and received LAK infusions on days 12-14; but, the maintenance phase consisted of a *lower* IL-2 dose (2×10^6 U/m^2/day) given for a *longer* period of time (days 10-19). Ten patients with clinical characteristics comparable to those of patients in the previous study have been treated to date on this ongoing trial. The toxicity associated with the maintenance IL-2 was significantly reduced. Four of 9 patients responded: one had a CR for 5+ months, and three experienced PR for 11+, 6+ and 5+ months. Overall, the results of the three trials suggest that a higher dose of IL-2 is more effective than a lower dose. Moreover, if additional patients and longer follow-up validate the preliminary results of the current trial, a role for a longer IL-2 maintenance phase will be suggested.

In patients treated with IL-2 plus LAK cells, the contribution, if any, of ex-vivo-generated LAK cells to the tumor responses observed has not been established. In the largest randomized trial[30] 30-35% of patients with metastatic renal cell carcinoma responded to IL-2 plus LAK cells as well as to IL-2 alone, but the incidence of *complete* responses was somewhat higher with IL-2 plus LAK. In other randomized trials, the overall response rates with IL-2 plus LAK cells have been so low that the question could not possibly be tested.[32,35]

Cellular Immunotherapy After Bone Marrow Transplantation for Hematologic Malignancies

High-dose chemoradiotherapy and bone marrow transplantation (BMT) offer the possibility of cure for some patients with refractory acute leukemia or lymphoma.[26,27,39-42] Success, however, is limited by a very high relapse rate after BMT.[40-42] The systemic administration of IL-2 with or without reinfusion of ex vivo-generated LAK cells[26,39] represents a new potentially non-cross-resistant treatment modality for use as an adjunct to chemoradiotherapy and BMT as a way to eradicate the minimal residual disease, and thereby prevent or delay occurrence of relapses. This possibility is suggested by the following observations: 1) human leukemia and lymphoma cells are lysable by LAK cells in vitro[18,20,43]; 2) IL-2/LAK therapy has induced remissions in some patients with leukemia and lymphoma[26,30,44-48]; and 3) minimal residual disease, ie, complete remission, is readily attainable with present chemoradiotherapy pretransplant conditioning regimens. Although the rationale for using IL-2 ± LAK cells after BMT applies to both allogeneic and autologous BMT, initially the main focus has been on studies after autologous BMT (ABMT) because it represents a simpler clinical setting without the complications potentially posed by immunologic barriers between marrow donor and recipient. Moreover, immunotherapy after ABMT should, theoretically, be able to eradicate whatever clonogenic malignant cells might be present and reinfused with the stored marrow, thereby obviating the need for purging marrow of tumor cells.

Since relapses most often occur within the first year after ABMT,[40-42] IL-2 ± LAK cells would have to be administered early after ABMT, after the patients have recovered from ABMT-related toxicities, and at a time when the tumor burden is still minimal but before relapses are likely to have occured. On the assumption that IL-2-responsive LAK precursor cells must be present in order for IL-2/LAK therapy to be effective, we first investigated the reconstitution of IL-2-responsive LAK precursor activity in the circulation of patients after ABMT. The results showed that such activity is reconstituted as early as 17 days after ABMT.[49]

Second, the possibility was considered that patients would be extremely susceptible to IL-2 toxicity during the early posttransplant phase and might or might not respond immunologically to IL-2 administration. Therefore, a Phase Ib clinical trial with IL-2 alone was carried out after ABMT to identify the maximum tolerated dose of IL-2 and to document its immunomodulatory effects, if any.[50]

We administered IL-2 (Roche) by CIV infusion to 16 patients with acute leukemia or lymphoma 14 to 91 days (median 33) after ABMT. Patients were sequentially assigned to escalating IL-2 "induction" doses of 0.3-4.5 $\times 10^6$ U/m^2/day on days 1-5; Group I received 0.3×10^6 U/m^2/day, Group II 1.0×10^6 U/m^2/day, Group III 3.0×10^6 U/m^2/day and Group IV 4.5×10^6 U/m^2/day. After a rest period, all patients received a "maintenance" infusion of IL-2 at 0.3×10^6 U/m^2/day on days 12-21. All patients received induction IL-2 as inpatients. All patients completed the maintenance phase, usually as outpatients. The results are detailed elsewhere.[50]

Hematologic toxicities were limited to a transient decrease in the platelet counts with increased platelet transfusion requirements. Dose-limiting toxicities were hypotension and thrombocytopenia. All toxicities reversed quickly after IL-2 treatment was stopped.

Hematologic and immunologic tests were performed on day 0 (before IL-2 therapy) and day 7 (24 hours after completing the induction course), and on day 12 and day 23 (at the beginning and end of the maintenance phase). Neutrophil counts tended to rise throughout the course of IL-2 treatment.

All groups exhibited transient early lymphopenia followed by a rebound lymphocytosis 24 hours after finishing the IL-2 "induction" course. The count was significantly elevated over baseline in Groups II and III. Mean lymphocyte counts subsequently decreased but remained elevated above pretreatment values throughout the maintenance phase in all groups. Variable increases in the number of cells expressing CD3, CD4, CD8 and CD25 were observed on day 7.

IL-2 therapy increased the percentage of circulating lymphocytes expressing CD16 and CD56 surface markers which are associated with NK and LAK activities.

Peripheral blood lymphocytes were also tested serially for NK and LAKe activities. All patients tested had low levels of spontaneous LAKe on day 0. Group III patients exhibited an increase in both NK and LAKe activity but Groups I and II did not.

To determine whether LAKp activity would be augmented by IL-2 "induction," cells obtained on day 0 and day 7 were cultured for 5 days in IL-2 and then tested for lysis of Daudi cells. Nine of 10 patients tested had substantially increased LAKp activity. No statistically significant differences were noted between patient groups in this assay.

Thus, we have identified an IL-2 regimen that can be tolerated safely during the first few weeks after ABMT and induced immunomodulatory effects that appear to be dose-related. The toxicities and immunologic changes were somewhat similar to those reported in two other trials with different regimens and sources of IL-2.[51,52] Based on our results, we have initiated a Phase II trial of IL-2 (at the maximum tolerated dose) plus LAK cells in an attempt to reduce the relapse rate of lymphoma patients after ABMT.

We have initiated a similar set of studies in high risk relapse patients who have undergone *allogeneic* BMT for hematologic malignancies. The rationale is the same as that for using cellular immunotherapy after *autologous* BMT. The intent is that such therapy would induce or amplify a graft-vs-leukemia (GVL) effect exerted by cells from the infused foreign donor marrow. The principal potential complication is the induction or exacerbation of severe graft-vs-host disease (GVHD).

In animal models, the GVL effect may or may not be separable or distinguishable from the GVH reaction in that the effector cells responsible for the GVL effect and for GVHD have been the same in some models but different in others. Effector cells that mediate the GVL effect in animals and humans may include: 1) cytotoxic T lymphocytes (CTL) specific for minor histocompatibility antigens present on both normal host tissue and leukemic cells and/or against antigens expressed only or preferentially on malignant cells, 2) lymphocytes that mediate their antitumor effects via secondary lymphokine secretion and/or 3) cytolytic T or non-T cells that mediate their antitumor effect through an MHC-unrestricted mechanism. IL-2 can stimulate the proliferation and function of all the above-mentioned effector cells.

In murine models, IL-2 can induce, exacerbate or even protect against GVHD, depending on the model and the timing.[53,54,55] Little is known about the effect of LAK cells on GVHD. In one model, lethal GVHD was prevented by the addition of recipient-type "veto" LAK cells but was exacerbated by LAK cells of donor or third-party origin.[56]

The role of IL-2 or LAK in the GVL effect has received too little attention in murine models. In a syngeneic BMT model for lymphoma, IL-2 was curative.[57] In another syngeneic model, BMT using marrow activated by preincubation with IL-2 and followed by systemic administration of IL-2 reduced the number of metastases of melanoma[58] and cured some leukemic mice.[59] Finally, in one H2-incompatible BMT model, IL-2 administered at the time of BMT induced a significant GVL effect against a lymphoma, without exacerbating GVHD.[53,54] The results all suggest a graft-vs-tumor effect induced by IL-2 ± LAK cells.

Lymphocytes from patients who have undergone allogeneic BMT, when cultured in IL-2, can acquire LAK activity and lyse host tumor. Thus, LAKe cells from 20 of 33 allogeneic marrow recipients lysed host CML cells; in 22 of 37 cases the LAK cells also lysed HLA-disparate CML cells.[19] The lysis was mediated predominantly by cells of activated NK phenotype with a small fraction being CD3+ T cells. The LAK activity was inducible in cells from recipients of both T-cell-depleted and T-cell-replete marrow, and both in the presence or absence of GVHD. The authors concluded that an MHC unrestricted GVL effect was inducible in vitro after allogeneic BMT and that the use of IL-2/LAK cells after BMT might reduce the risk of relapse.

There is cogent circumstantial clinical evidence for the existence of a GVL effect in vivo after allogeneic BMT.[60,61] This evidence can be summarized as follows: 1) the incidence of leukemic relapse is lower after allogeneic than after syngeneic BMT, 2) the incidence of leukemic relapse is lower in allogeneic marrow recipients who develop acute and/or chronic GVHD than in allogeneic marrow recipients who do not develop GVHD, 3) the incidence of leukemic relapse is lower in recipients of allogeneic marrow without GVHD than it is in recipients of syngeneic marrow, 4) the incidence of leukemic relapse is higher in recipients of T-cell depleted allogeneic marrow than in recipients of unmodified allogeneic marrow and 5) cases of a temporal association between a flare-up of GVHD and disease remission have been reported. IL-2/LAK therapy, therefore, may be a particularly appropriate form of consolidative therapy after allogeneic BMT for hematologic malignancies because it might induce or amplify a GVL effect. A Phase Ib trial of IL-2 has already been initiated with a view to a subsequent therapy trial of IL-2 plus LAK cells to decrease relapse rates after allogeneic BMT. Substantial results should be generated within the next 2 years.

Clinical Cellular Immunotherapy Using Tumor-Specific T Lymphocytes

Murine studies[4] suggest that immune T cells have several theoretical advantages over LAK cells, including: 1) target specificity, 2) ability to "home" to sites of tumor and proliferate there in response to tumor, 3) ability to persist in vivo long-term, 4) ability to maintain proliferative and cytolytic function in the presence of far lower IL-2 concentration and 5) immunologic memory.

Many attempts have been made to detect T cells specifically reactive to autologous tumors in humans. The most encouraging results have been reported with T cells obtained from biopsies of melanoma—designated as tumor-infiltrating lymphocytes (TILs)—and grown in IL-2. In a variable percentage of cases such cells expressed specific cytolytic reactivity for autologous tumor cells.[62,63] Preliminary results of the first clinical trial using cyclophosphamide, TILs and a short course of high-dose IL-2 for patients with metastatic melanoma suggested that 50% of the patients who received the full treatment exhibited a partial response.[64]

The encouraging tumor responses represent a major impetus to further laboratory and clinical studies to confirm, extend and improve the results. A number of practical problems remain. Only 20 of the 40 patients in the trial reported[64] actually received the TIL cells, partly because the disease is so virulent that patients deteriorated clinically during the weeks required for TIL generation and became ineligible for the treatment and because, for reasons not clear, TILs from a substantial proportion of tumor biopsies did not grow to adequate numbers.

During the past 2 years we have been generating TILs from melanoma biopsies, expanding them in IL-2 and characterizing them phenotypically and functionally in terms of autologous tumor lysis. The results,[65] summarized below, demonstrate that TILs can be grown to large number in approximately 60% of cases, that they are overwhelmingly $CD3^+$ $CD8^+$, and that in the overwhelming majority of cases the cultured TILs specifically or preferentially lyse autologous but not allogeneic melanoma in a Class I MHC-restricted fashion.[65]

Culture of Tumor-Infiltrating Lymphocytes

Tumor biopsies were obtained from subcutaneous nodules or lymph nodes of patients with metastatic melanoma. Tumor cells were finely minced and gently forced through stainless steel mesh into complete media, which consisted of AIM V supplemented with L-glutamine (2 mM), streptomycin sulfate (50 µg/mL) and gentamicin sulfate (10 µg/mL). Cultures were initiated in complete media supplemented with 1000 U/mL r-IL-2 (Hoffman-LaRoche, Nutley, NJ) and/or r-IL-4 1000 U/mL (Immunex, Seattle, WA) at a concentration of 0.5-1.0×10^6 mononuclear cells/mL. Aliquots of tumor cells and TILs were cryopreserved in liquid nitrogen in a solution of 10% DMSO and 90% fetal calf serum. Cultures were begun in either 24-well plates or 75-cm^2 flasks (Corning Glass Works, Corning, NY) and incubated at 37 C in 5% CO_2. Cultures were counted and refed every 3-4 days in complete media with the lymphokine(s). Subsequently, cultures were transferred to and grown in 750-cm culture bags (Baxter/Fenwal, Deerfield, IL).

TIL cells were assayed for lytic activity at multiple times during their growth, using a standard 4-hour ^{51}Cr release assay. Various targets were used, including thawed "fresh" autologous and allogeneic melanoma cells (cryopreserved when the tumor was processed), when available.

Growth and Phenotype of TIL in IL-2

Some TILs were expanded to $>10^{11}$ cells. However, in about 40% of biopsies cells do not grow to large number, either because there are not enough lymphocytes in the initial tumor specimens or for other unknown reasons. A 14-24,000-fold expansion was observed in 15/18 TIL cultures. With time in culture, there is a progressive increase in $CD3^+$ cells with a very marked increase in the percent $CD8^+$ cells.

Lytic Activity of TILs

At various times in culture, TILs were tested for their ability to lyse autologous tumor, allogeneic melanoma cells, K562 (the NK target) and

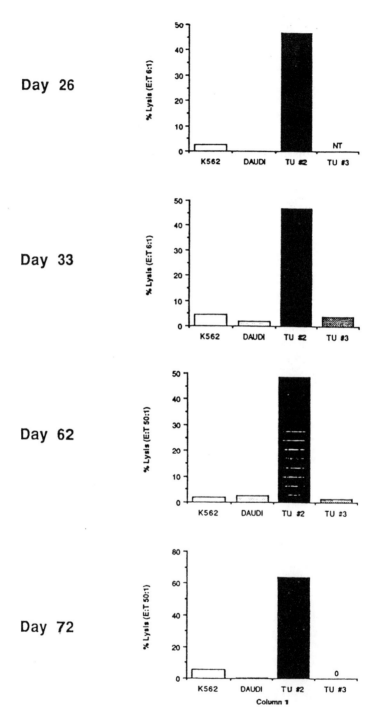

Figure 8-2. TILs from patient 2 were grown in IL-2 and serially tested in a ^{51}Cr-release assay for lysis of autologous tumors (TU2) versus an allogeneic melanoma (TU3), K562 and Daudi.

Daudi. (the LAK cell target). Figure 8-2 shows that TILs from Patient 2 tested from day 26 to day 72 in culture significantly lysed the autologous tumor (TU2) but not any of the other targets. Criss-cross experiments demonstrate that the allogeneic melanoma (which was not lysed) can, in fact, be lysed specifically by its own TILs. Specific lysis of autologous tumor without concurrent lysis of allogeneic melanoma was observed in 11/14 TIL cultures tested. The autologous tumor lysis is MHC Class I-restricted. The lysis can be blocked by antibody directed at Class I determinants but not against Class II determinants or by other control antibodies.[65]

TIL Clinical Trial

Kawakame et al[66] have reported that IL-4 can, at times, preferentially enhance the growth of cells with specific autologous reactivity. Although this is not a consistent or reproducible finding, some of our laboratory results were supportive. Therefore, a clinical trial has been initiated for patients with metastatic malignant melanoma using cyclophosphamide plus TILs grown in a combination of Roche IL-2 (1000 U/mL) and Sterling IL-4 (1000 U/mL), plus systemic IL-2. The protocol will consist of: 1) IV cyclophosphamide at 25 mg/kg, 2) intravenous infusion of the patients' autologous TILs given 36 hours after the cyclophosphamide and 3) a 10-day CIV infusion of IL-2 at a dose of 2×10^6 U/m^2/day beginning at the time of administration of the TILs. Those patients from whose tumor TILs fail to grow or who do not have accessible tumor for TIL generation are being treated with cytoxan and IL-2 without any TILs. The study is designed to determine the toxicity, in vivo immunomodulation and objective response rate of this approach. An additional objective is the phenotypic and functional immunologic characterization of the TILs generated. The trial is in progress. Substantial results are anticipated within a year.

Conclusions and Directions

Cellular immunotherapy is receiving a great deal of investigative attention, both in experimental models and in clinical trials. Most of the attention has focused on the use of IL-2 with LAK cells or T lymphocytes with putative tumor-specific reactivity.

Although the usefulness of IL-2/LAK therapy remains controversial, there is no question whatsoever that IL-2 ± LAK cells can cause the partial or complete regression of grossly apparent, measurable cancer in *some* patients, sometimes for years. Such regressions, achieved without cytotoxic chemotherapy, radiation or surgery, must be considered especially significant because they represent the first evidence of efficacy of a purely biologic approach to cancer therapy. Moreover, the results were obtained with a regimen that was largely empirically derived and a treatment modality whose antitumor effect is mediated by mechanisms that are still unknown. One can, therefore, hope that once a more rational or optimal regimen is identified and more is learned about the underlying mechanism by which this treatment mediates tumor regression, better results will be obtained with less toxicity and greater antitumor efficacy.

Several issues have been identified that must be resolved by well-designed laboratory and clinical studies. It is necessary to identify by some laboratory or clinical parameters those patients who are most likely to respond and those least likely to respond to such therapy so as to spare the latter group the treatment-associated toxicity and focus on improving the therapeutic index for the former group. The contribution, if any, of the exogenously generated LAK cells to the therapeutic effects observed must be determined. This can be achieved only in prospectively randomized trials to compare IL-2 alone with IL-2 plus LAK cells in a clinical setting in which treatment with IL-2 plus LAK cells induces a substantial response rate, eg, ≥40%. If the response rate is low, the question is neither interesting, nor significant, nor practically testable in any reasonable number of patients. Should exogenous LAK cells be found not to contribute to the therapeutic efficacy, then the cumbersome and costly technology associated with their generation could be eliminated and emphasis could be placed on combining IL-2 with other lymphokines or cytokines or monoclonal antibodies in vivo. On the other hand, should ex-vivo-generated LAK cells be demonstrated to contribute significantly to the therapeutic effect, then emphasis will be placed on identifying the requisite effector cell subset and exploring other ways to enhance or augment the large-scale generation of the requisite cell in vitro and/or in vivo by using other cytokines, eg, interferons and/or lymphokines such as IL-4[67] and/or other activation factors such as antibodies.[68]

IL-2/LAK therapy has usually been administered as a single course and has induced largely partial responses. Once optimal and less toxic regimens are developed, several courses of treatment will be possible and a higher rate of complete tumor regressions may be induced. Moreover, IL-2/LAK therapy has been used alone as an alternative to chemotherapy, ie, either in patients with types of cancers for which no effective conventional therapy is available or in patients who have failed to respond to other available therapies. In the future, immunotherapy is likely to be used in conjunction with other known treatment modalities. The studies described using IL-2/LAK therapy after BMT represent one example of such combination therapy.

LAK cell generation for clinical use is now automated and adapted to commercially available closed-system disposable plasticware, with a resultant improvement in safety and a decrease in cost and labor. All our studies have involved leukaphereses performed with a closed-system continuous flow cell separator (CS-3000, Baxter Healthcare Corporation, Deerfield,

IL). Flow rates of 40-60 mL/minute and 4-hour collections have resulted in mean values of 5.2×10^{10} lymphocytes per collection, or 4.3×10^9 lymphocytes per liter of blood processed. This represents over 80% efficiency.

Theoretically, the leukaphereses can be readily performed at a blood bank. The only limitation is the clinical state of the patient, which is, unfortunately, often precarious. Indeed, the regimens of IL-2/LAK that have been most therapeutic have also been most toxic with major hemodynamic changes, hypotension, oliguria and fluid overload with potential compromise of respiratory function. Although the toxicities are always readily reversible on stopping IL-2, the clinical status of most patients would probably prohibit them from being managed at a blood bank. It is very possible, however, that less toxic regimens will be developed in the future; the aphereses could then be performed at a blood bank. The in vitro LAK cell generation and the harvesting for infusion can be performed at a blood bank if the requisite incubators and computerized automix machinery are available.

The potential use of tumor-specific T cells for cancer therapy, though extremely well-explored in animal models, remains a formidable problem in humans. The encouraging preliminary results of TIL therapy for melanoma[64] must be confirmed, extended and improved. The optimal IL-2 regimen, ie, dose, route and duration, needs to be identified. Since even TILs from melanoma biopsies, which have been studied the most, often fail to grow to adequate numbers, better conditions for their expansion must be identified. This may involve other T-cell activation signals, including lymphokines, monoclonal antibodies and/or putative tumor antigens. Although studies are already in progress with TIL transfected with the gene for the production of tumor necrosis factor, the effector cell subset that mediates the therapeutic results has not yet been identified. That would require a clinical trial in which a particular subset is obtained by positive or negative selection, characterized phenotypically and functionally for tumor-specific reactivity and then infused. Alternatively and less satisfactorily, identification could be made by obtaining circumstantial evidence in the form of retrospective correlation between the characteristics of the TILs infused and the clinical response. Large clinical trials with a substantial clinical tumor response rate would be required.

Although the bulk of the laboratory evidence for the existence of tumor-specific T cells in humans and the only preliminary evidence for their therapeutic efficacy have been derived from studies in patients with malignant melanoma, some of the findings or principles might be applicable to patients with other malignancies. For example, T cells reactive to the idiotype of a particular B-cell lymphoma or to the protein product of some mutated oncogene could, conceivably, be generated, identified, expanded, cloned and eventually infused for therapy. Should advances in our knowledge make that possible, it is likely that such exquisitely tumor-specific T-cell therapy will also be used not as the sole modality but in combination with other therapies. Thus, past progress and present status provide grounds for optimism regarding the potential of cellular immunotherapy for cancer—a potential that will be realized by a collaborative mix of basic laboratory research and clinical trials.

References

1. Fefer A, Cheever M, Greenberg P. Overview of prospects and problems of lymphocyte transfer for cancer therapy. In: Fefer A, Goldstein AL, eds. Progress in cancer research and therapy: The potential role of T cells in cancer therapy. New York: Raven Press, 1982:1-6.
2. Fefer A, Cheever M, Greenberg P. Lymphocyte transfer as potential cancer immunotherapy. In: Mihich E, ed. Immunological approaches to cancer therapeutics. New York: John Wiley & Sons, Inc., 1982:299-332.
3. Fefer A, Einstein A Jr, Cheever M, Berenson J. Models for syngeneic adoptive chemoimmunotherapy of murine leukemias. Ann NY Acad Sci 1976;276:573-83.
4. Greenberg P. Adoptive T cell therapy of tumors: Mechanisms operative in the recognition and elimination of tumor cells. In: Dixon F, ed. Advances in immunology. Orlando, FL: Academic Press, Inc., 1991;28:355.
5. Fass L, Fefer A. Studies of adoptive chemoimmunotherapy of a Friend virus-induced lymphoma. Cancer Res 1972;32:997-1001.
6. Greenberg P, Cheever M, Fefer A. Eradication of disseminated murine leukemia by chemo-immunotherapy with cyclophosphamide and adoptively transferred immune syngeneic Lyt-1^+2^- T lymphocytes. J Exp Med 1981;154:952-63.
7. Greenberg P. Therapy of murine leukemia with cyclophosphamide and immune Lyt-2^+ cells: Cytolytic T cells can mediate eradication of disseminated leukemia. J Immunol 1986;136:1917-22.
8. Cheever M, Greenberg P, Fefer A, Gillis S. Augmentation of the anti-tumor therapeutic efficacy of long-term cultured T lymphocytes by in vivo administration of purified interleukin-2. J Exp Med 1982; 155;968.
9. Ortaldo JR, Mason A, Overton R. Lymphokine-activated killer cells. J Exp Med 1986;164:1193-205.
10. Rosenberg S, Mulé J, Spiess P, et al. Regression of established pulmonary metastases and subcutaneous tumor mediated by the systemic administration of high-dose recombinant interleukin 2. J Exp Med 1985;161:1168-88.
11. Mulé J, Shu S, Rosenberg S. The anti-tumor efficacy of lymphokine-activated killer cells and recombinant interleukin 2 in vivo. J Immunol 1985;135:646-52.

12. Lafreniere R, Rosenberg S. Successful immunotherapy of murine experimental hepatic metastases with lymphokine-activated killer cells and recombinant interleukin-2. Cancer Res 1985;45:3735-41.

13. Mazumder A, Rosenberg S. Successful immunotherapy of natural killer-resistant established pulmonary melanoma metastases by the intravenous adoptive transfer of syngeneic lymphocytes activated in vitro by interleukin 2. J Exp Med 1984;159:495-507.

14. Sondel P, Hank J, Kohler P, et al. Destruction of autologous human lymphocytes by interleukin-2-activated cytotoxic cells. J Immunol 1986;137:502-11.

15. Grimm E, Wilson D. The human lymphokine-activated killer system. IV. Purified recombinant interleukin-2 activates cytotoxic lymphocytes which lyse both natural killer-resistant autologous and allogeneic tumors and Trinitrophenyl-modified autologous peripheral blood lymphocytes. Cell Immunol 1985;94:568-78.

16. Lotzová E, Ades E. Natural killer cells: Definition, heterogeneity, lytic mechanism, functions and clinical application. Nat Immun Cell Growth Regul 1989;8:1-9.

17. Robertson MJ, Ritz J. Biology and clinical relevance of human natural killer cells. Blood 1990;76:2421-38.

18. Lotzová E, Savary CA, Herberman RB. Induction of NK cell activity against fresh human leukemia in culture with interleukin 2. J Immunol 1987;138:2718-27.

19. Mackinnon S, Hows JM, Goldman JM. Induction of in vitro graft-versus-leukemia activity following bone marrow transplantation for chronic myeloid leukemia. Blood 1990;76:2037-45.

20. Oshimi K, Oshimi Y, Akutsu M, et al. Cytotoxicity of interleukin 2-activated lymphocytes for leukemia and lymphoma cells. Blood 1986;68:938-48.

21. Dawson MM, Johnston D, Taylor GM, Moore M. Lymphokine activated killing of fresh human leukaemias. Leuk Res 1986;10:683-8.

22. Landay AL, Zarcone D, Grossi CE, Bauer K. Relationship between target cell cycle and susceptibility to natural killer lysis. Cancer Res 1987;47:2767-70.

23. Allavena P, Damia G, Colombo T, et al. Lymphokine-activated killer (LAK) and monocyte-mediated cytotoxicity on tumor cell lines resistant to antitumor agents. Cell Immunol 1989;120:250-8.

24. Lista P, Fierro MT, Liao X-S, et al. Lymphokine-activated killer (LAK) cells inhibit the clonogenic growth of human leukemic stem cells. Eur J Haematol 1989;42:425-30.

25. Lotzová E, Savary CA, Herberman RB. Inhibition of clonogenic growth of fresh leukemia cells by unstimulated and IL-2 stimulated NK cells of normal donors. Leuk Res 1987;11:1059-66.

26. West WH, Tauer KW, Yannelli JR, et al. Constant-infusion recombinant interleukin-2 in adoptive immunotherapy of advanced cancer. N Engl J Med 1987;316:898-905.

27. Rosenberg SA, Lotze MT, Muul LM, et al. A progress report on the treatment of 157 patients with advanced cancer using lymphokine-activated killer cells and interleukin-2 or high-dose interleukin-2 alone. N Engl J Med 1987;316:889-97.

28. Thompson JA, Lee DJ, Lindgren CG, et al. Influence of schedule of interleukin 2 administration on therapy with interleukin-2 and lymphokine activated killer cells. Cancer Res 1989;49:235-40.

29. Thompson J, Collins C, Higuchi C, et al. High-dose continuous intravenous infusion interleukin-2 and lymphokine-activated killer cell therapy for renal cell carcinoma (abstract). In: Proceedings of the AACR. Philadelphia: American Association for Cancer Research, 1990:271.

30. Rosenberg SA, Lotze MT, Yang JC, et al. Experience with the use of high-dose interleukin-2 in the treatment of 652 cancer patients. Ann Surg 1989;210:474-85.

31. Fisher RI, Coltman CA Jr, Doroshow JH, et al. Metastatic renal cancer treated with interleukin-2 and lymphokine-activated killer cells. Ann Intern Med 1988;18:518-23.

32. McCabe M, Stablein D, Hawkins M. The modified Group C experience—Phase III randomized trials of IL-2 vs IL-2/LAK in advanced renal cell carcinoma and advanced melanoma (abstract). Philadelphia: American Society of Clinical Oncology, 1991:213.

33. Thompson JA, Lee DJ, Lindgren CG, et al. Influence of dose and duration of infusion of interleukin-2 on toxicity and immunomodulation. J Clin Oncol 1988;6:669-78.

34. Margolin KA, Rayner A, Hawkins MJ, et al. Interleukin-2 and lymphokine-activated killer cell therapy of solid tumors: Analysis of toxicity and management guidelines. J Clin Oncol 1989;7:486-98.

35. Rosenberg S. Immunotherapy of cancer by systemic administration of lymphoid cells and IL-2. J Biol Resp Mod 1984;3:501.

36. Thompson JA, Lee DJ, Cox WW, et al. Recombinant interleukin-2 toxicity, pharmacokinetics, and immunomodulatory effects in a phase I trial. Cancer Res 1987;47:4202-07.

37. Parkinson D. Interleukin-2 in cancer therapy. Semin Oncol 1988; 15:10-26.

38. Thompson J, Benyunes M, Benz L, et al. Prolonged continuous intravenous (CIV) infusion interleukin-2 and lymphokine-activated killer (LAK) cell therapy for renal carcinoma (abstract). Philadelphia: American Society of Clinical Oncology, 1991:179.

39. Rosenberg S, Lotze M, Muul L, et al. Observations on the systemic administration of autologous lymphokine-activated killer cells and recombinant interleukin-2 to patients with metastatic cancer. N Engl J Med 1985;313:1485-92.

40. Petersen F, Appelbaum F, Hill R, et al. Autologous marrow transplantation for malignant lymphoma: A report of 101 cases from Seattle. J Clin Oncol 1990;8:638-47.

41. Philip T, Armitage J, Spitzer G, et al. High dose therapy and autologous bone marrow transplantation after failure of conventional chemotherapy in adults with intermediate grade or high grade non-Hodgkin's lymphoma. N Engl J Med 1987;316:1493-8.
42. Takvorian T, Canellos G, Ritz J, et al. Prolonged disease-free survival after autologous bone marrow transplantation in patients with non-Hodgkin's lymphoma with a poor prognosis. N Engl J Med 1987; 316:1499-505.
43. Adler A, Chervenick P, Whiteside T, et al. Interleukin-2 induction of lymphokine-activated killer (LAK) activity in the peripheral blood and bone marrow of acute leukemia patients. I. Feasibility of LAK generation in adult patients with active disease and in remission. Blood 1988;71:709-16.
44. Paciucci PA, Holland JF, Glidewell O, Odchimar R. Recombinant interleukin-2 by continuous infusion and adoptive transfer of recombinant interleukin-2-activated cells in patients with advanced cancer. J Clin Oncol 1989;7:869-78.
45. Schoof DD, Gramolini BA, Davidson DL, et al. Adoptive immunotherapy of human cancer using low-dose recombinant interleukin-2 and lymphokine-activated killer cells. Cancer Res 1988;48:5007-10.
46. Bernstein ZP, Vaickus L, Friedman N, et al. IL-2 LAK therapy of non-Hodgkin's lymphoma and Hodgkin's disease. J Immunother 1991;10:141-6.
47. Foa R, Melone G, Tosti S, et al. Treatment of acute myeloid leukemia patients with recombinant IL2: Clinical and biological findings (abstract). Blood 1990;76(10,Suppl 1):270a.
48. Foa R, Meloni G, Tosti S, et al. Treatment of residual disease in acute leukemia patients with recombinant interleukin 2 (IL2): Clinical and biological findings. Bone Marrow Transplant 1990;6:98-102.
49. Higuchi AM, Thompson JA, Cox T, et al. Lymphokine-activated killer function following autologous bone marrow transplantation for refractory hematological malignancies. Cancer Res 1989;49:5509-13.
50. Higuchi CM, Thompson JA, Petersen FB, et al. Toxicity and immunomodulatory effects of interleukin-2 after autologous bone marrow transplantation for hematologic malignancies. Blood 1991:(in press).
51. Gottlieb DJ, Brenner MK, Heslop HE, et al. A phase I clinical trial of recombinant interleukin 2 following high dose chemo-radiotherapy for haematological malignancy: Applicability to the elimination of minimal residual disease. Br J Cancer 1989;60:610-15.
52. Blaise D, Olive D, Stoppa AM, et al. Hematologic and immunologic effects of the systemic administration of recombinant interleukin-2 after autologous bone marrow transplantation. Blood 1990;76:1092-97.

53. Sykes M, Romick ML, Sachs DH. Interleukin-2 prevents graft-versus-host disease while preserving the graft-versus-leukemia effect of allogeneic T cells. Proc Natl Acad Sci USA 1990;87:5633-7.

54. Sykes M, Romick ML, Hoyles KA, Sachs DH. In vivo administration of interleukin-2 plus T cell-depleted syngeneic marrow prevents graft-versus-host disease mortality and permits alloengraftment. J Exp Med 1990;171:645-58.

55. Sprent J, Schaefer M, Gao E-K, Korngold R. Role of T cell subsets in lethal graft-versus-host disease (GVHD) directed to class I versus class II H-2 differences. J Exp Med 1988;167:556-69.

56. Azuma E, Yamamoto H, Kaplan J. Use of lymphokine-activated killer cells to prevent bone marrow graft rejection and lethal graft-vs-host disease. J Immunol 1989;143:1524-9.

57. Slavin S, Eckerstein A, Weiss L. Adoptive immunotherapy in conjunction with bone marrow transplantation—amplification of natural host defence mechanisms against cancer by recombinant IL-2. Nat Immun Cell Growth Regul 1988;7:180-4.

58. Agah R, Malloy B, Kerner M, et al. Potent graft antitumor effect in natural killer-resistant disseminated tumors by transplantation of interleukin 2-activated syngeneic bone marrow in mice. Cancer Res 1989;49:5959-63.

59. Charak BS, Brynes RK, Groshen S, et al. Bone marrow transplantation with interleukin-2-activated bone marrow followed by interleukin-2 therapy for acute myeloid leukemia in mice. Blood 1990; 76:2187-90.

60. Sullivan K, Weiden P, Storb R, et al. Influence of acute and chronic graft-versus-host disease on relapse and survival after bone marrow transplantation from HLA-identical siblings as treatment of acute and chronic leukemia. Blood 1989;73:1720-8.

61. Fefer A, Truitt RL, Sullivan KM. Adoptive cellular therapy: Graft-vs-tumor responses after bone marrow transplantation. In: DeVita V, Hellman S, Rosenberg SA, eds. Biologic therapy of cancer: Principles and practice. Philadelphia: JB Lippincott Co., 1991:237-46.

62. Topalian S, Solomon D, Rosenberg S.Tumor-specific cytolysis by lymphocytes infiltrating human melanoma. J Immunol 1989;142: 3714-25.

63. Itoh K, Platsoucas C, Balch C. Autologous tumor-specific cytotoxic T lymphocytes in the infiltrate of human metastatic melanomas: Activation by interleukin-2 and autologous tumor cells, and involvement of the T cell receptor. J Exp Med 1988;168:1419-41.

64. Rosenberg S, Packard B, Aebersold P, et al. Use of tumor-infiltrating lymphocytes and interleukin-2 in the immunotherapy of patients with metastatic melanoma: A preliminary report. N Engl J Med 1988:319:1676-80.

65. Higuchi C, Triesman J, Thompson J, et al. Cytolytic T-lymphocytes infiltrating human melanoma expanded by culture with interleukin-

2 (abstract) In: Proceedings of the AACR. Philadelphia: American Association for Cancer Research, 1990:269.

66. Kawakame Y, Rosenberg SA, Lotze MT. Interleukin-4 promotes the growth of tumor-infiltrating lymphocytes cytotoxic for human autologous melanoma. J Exp Med 1988;168:2183-91.

67. Higuchi C, Thompson J, Lindgren C, et al. Induction of lymphokine-activated killer activity by interleukin-4 in human lymphocytes pre-activated by interleukin-2 in vivo or in vitro. Cancer Res 1989; 49:6487-92.

68. Treisman J, Higuchi C, Thompson J, et al. Interleukin-4 enhances the proliferation of lymphocytes from IL-2-treated cancer patients induced by IL-2 or mitogenic antibodies. Cancer Res 1990;50:1160-4.

Index